PHARMACY MOVEMENT

How to Prescribe Social and Digital Medicines

PROF. ARUN NADARASA

Foreword by Medical NLP Founder Garner Thomson

Warning—Disclaimer

The purpose of this book is to educate and entertain.

The author and/or publisher do not guarantee that anyone following these techniques, suggestions, tips, ideas, or strategies will become successful. The author and/or publisher shall have neither liability nor responsibility to anyone with respect to any loss or damage caused, or alleged to be caused, directly or indirectly by the information contained in this book.

DEDICATION

This book is dedicated to all the community pharmacists in UK who love their profession and who strive to improve the health and wellbeing of their patients by enhancing the use of Social and Digital Prescribing within community pharmacies.

When I realised that both my dance and pharmacy background could be combined for the benefit of my patients, I was inspired to start this book to share my message. This happened when I was sitting at the RPS Conference in 2016 – at the IIC in Birmingham – where I first heard of the NHS 5 Year Forward View. There was a need to bridge the gap between health and wellbeing.

I sincerely hope this book will inspire you to become involved in this blue ocean within the pharmacy sector.

Love
Arun Nadarasa

Contents

Reviews of
Pharmacy Movement

"The mind and body are irrevocably connected, and a balance between the two is essential to maintain an intricate harmony. Being a medic alongside a musician and artist, I have incorporated the benefits of the creative arts into my clinical practice to complement medication management and support quality of life. I would see Arun's efforts as a commendable start towards a combined philosophy within UK pharmacies. It has great potential to lend itself to scientifically validated studies as it evolves."

Dr Ramya Mohan, MB BS, MRCPsych Medical Director and Head, I MANAS London Senior Consultant Child and Adolescent Psychiatrist, Medical Educator, Musician, Artist & Author

"Engaging and enjoyable. Arun brings forth a whole new way of looking at health and wellbeing in *Pharmacy Movement*. This produces a methodical approach, which makes this book not only an easy read, but also thought-provoking. It can turn you from being an employee to a pharmapreneur."

Kwame Osei, Founder of European Buck Session, World Championship of Krump Dance

"Arun wrote this book so that you can create new services in your community pharmacy. A superb demonstration on how this blue ocean can have a profound positive impact in the health and wellbeing of patients. *Pharmacy Movement* is the key to unlocking the immense potential that resides within each of us."

Marvin Munzu,
Media Pharmacist & Inspirational Speaker
Author of *Success Secrets 4 Students*

"Ever since I first met Arun, I have been struck by his seemingly singular desire to enrich the lives of those he feels he can help. Genius or delusional, I am still undecided."

Owynn Baker, Pharmacist Manager
Lloyds Pharmacy

"In this book, Arun opens your eyes to the benefits of activity for physical and mental wellbeing. It built on the concept of Healthy Living Pharmacy, and making every contact count through the conversation and action of Health Champions and Pharmacists."

Mike Holden, Company Director and Pharmacist
Pharmacy Complete

"Arun's book is a true gem; his insight is inspiring and revolutionary. Totally recommend it!"

Simone Sistarelli,
Dance Teacher Popping For Parkinson's

"Arun has thought very hard on bringing forward the future, and his idea of virtual consultation and movement will be the way forward. A good mix of interviews with leaders in their fields make for an excellent read."

Dr Talib Abubacker MBBS MRCGP Medical NLP
Master Practitioner

"The ability to use new technology in the community pharmacy setting is fundamental for this industry to push forward despite government cut backs in recent years."

Hirkirit Virdee, Company Director,
Pharmacist and Doctor
Pharmacy Blockchain

"Arun lays bare the untapped potential of creating SROI with clarity. There is nothing which will seem outside your reach after you read *Pharmacy Movement*. Everything appears as easy to digest information, you wonder why it didn't occur to you sooner. The secret to the book's appeal is its revolutionary concept."

Srishti Poojari, Lawyer and Krumper F.A.M.O.U.S
Fauj, Street Sisters & Desi Buck

"Dance meets Pharmacy, this book is a must have for all dancers wishing to improve the wellness of their local community through joint partnerships with pharmacists using social prescribing schemes. No more social isolation for the senior citizens!"

Bhagya Lakshmi, Company Director
Orphic Dance

"This book will move your mindset from scarcity to abundance as it will open your eyes to a new income stream, which is currently untapped within the pharmacy industry. This is a must-read book for all pharmacists."

Vishal Morjaria, Award Winning Author, International
Transformation Speaker, Coach
WOW Your Way To Wealth

"*Pharmacy Movement* is an incredible and revolutionary concept which I believe forms a robust new dimension in managing patient care. Arun very clearly outlines the benefits of non-pharmacological approaches in supporting our patients; medication is not always the answer to every disease."

Dr Kaniseya Kamalanathan, GP Trainee
Sports Advocate

About The Author

Arun wrote this book so that you can elevate your fulfilment in life. The author currently lives in the UK and is the founder of several start-ups. He has travelled internationally as a professional dance artist, as well as performing at Wembley SSE Arena in front of 10,000 people in April 2017.

Arun transformed his life by choosing to combine both his background in dance and his professional education, which culminated in *Pharmacy Movement*. He envisions Social & Digital Prescribing to become mainstream within the NHS and community pharmacies.

Acknowledgements

I would like to express my gratitude to Owynn Baker for supporting me in my journey to become an inspiring community pharmacist. He has always been there for me when I needed advice and is a role model for me. It is thanks to him that I have gained confidence over the years to finally write this book.

I also thank Robin Sharma for permanently altering my perception of life, it was his book "Lead Without A Title" which began my pursuit of personal development, which has had an immense impact in both my personal and professional life.

None of this would have been possible without my family who have always supported me in my dance career.

Finally, my most humble gratitude for the creators of Krump, Tight Eyez and Big Mijo which enabled me to express my feelings artistically when I needed it the most.

Foreword

Arun Nadarasa is the first person I have had the pleasure of training who has gone on to create a potentially life-changing field of his own.

The lives he sets out to change are the chronically ill, the aged, the sufferers of medically unexplained conditions—those dispossessed patients who do not fit the restrictions of today's time-poor, financially strapped tick-box culture of Western medicine.

A pharmacist who is seeking to find ways to minimise the over-prescription of, and over-dependence on, modern drugs is a rare beast. Even rarer is someone who has the vision and energy to offer alternatives to the knee-jerk response that has created the phenomenon of 'polypharmacy', the concurrent use of multiple medications, often with adverse effect on the patient.

Arun is such a pharmacist. But he is also a polymath with an unquenchable thirst for information and expertise. And, perhaps most important, he is a highly talented and innovative dancer, which—as recent research informs us—helps 'format' the brain to facilitate more rapid learning and increased creativity.

Arun has another rare gift: he doesn't know (or, perhaps, refuses to contemplate) what it is he is not supposed to be able to do. As a result, ideas, plans and projects erupt from his fertile imagination in breath-taking numbers and with breath-taking speed.

Of all his ideas, I am most in love with his concept of replacing an essentially palliative approach to healthcare with a succession of easily applicable preventive measures, including his annual 'stress inoculation'. This salutogenic, or health-supporting, approach is entirely aligned with Medical NLP's commitment to helping develop a world committed to actively pursuing healing and health, rather than simply managing disease.

I am honoured to be asked to write this foreword, and, also to be part of the birth of a system which I truly believe can add substantially to this aim.

—GARNER THOMSON LONDON 2017
Creator and Developer of Medical NLP
Neurolinguistic Programming
Master Practitioner and Master Trainer
Author of *Magic in Practice – Introducing Medical NLP,
the Art and Science of Language in Healing and Health*

The Time To Act Is Now

In the UK, the NHS has an allocated budget for community pharmacies. On the December 17th, 2015, it was announced that its budget will reduce by 6 percent by 2016 [1]. This led to a massive campaign by the NPA which gathered 2.2 million signatures [2]. Both the NPA and PSNC brought the government to court due to lack of communication and research with the sector, but the attempt was unsuccessful [3].

The NHS Five Year Forward View (5YFV) Document was released on October 22nd, 2014 [4] and was recently updated on March 31st, 2017 [5]. The document sets out recommendations to shift from a reactive approach to a pro-active approach in-order to reduce the severe challenges the NHS is facing. It emphasises the aim to bridge the health and wellbeing gap. There has been a shift to increase the number of Healthy Living Pharmacies (HLP) in the UK to help the sector meet that objective [6].

Currently, many newly qualified pharmacists are finding it difficult to find a full-time profession due to the lack of experience, and many locums are finding it harder to acquire regular shifts. Most notably, this is because there are 26 schools of pharmacy in England and the supply is far exceeding the demands of the market. With pharmacy cuts and the increasing number of candidates, the rate of pay for pharmacists has been drastically reduced, as well as being asked to do more services in return. As a result, many potential graduates feel discouraged to pursue this profession due to the direction it is heading in, which becomes apparent with the number of articles and comments made by current pharmacists and senior pharmacists online.

Social Prescribing
For The Win

Social Prescribing has been referred as 'signposting' in the community pharmacy, with no remuneration in delivering this specific service. It has been used over the past 30 years by pioneers such as the Bromley-By-Bow Centre [7] and many others which led to the establishment of the Social Prescribing Network (SPN) on March 9th 2016 [8]. At the Social Prescribing Network Annual Conference – which was held at The King's Fund on May 18th, 2017 – more than 400 delegates attended and the research results were very promising [9]. Additionally, Prince Charles was also present to show his support for social prescribing, however, he could not speak due to Purdah [10].

Up to 20 percent of GP appointments are for non-medical reasons [11] where Jeremy Hunt supports social prescribing. [12]. There are 1.8 million daily visits to 14,059 community pharmacies [13,14], with 44,000 pharmacists in this sector [15,16]. We are ideally placed to provide health and wellbeing services including Social & Digital Prescribing where MHRA has provided the CE marking for mobile apps meeting the correct standards [17,18]. The NHS also has a dedicated app store for those meeting the required criteria [19].

There are 44 STPs in UK [20] where 75 percent support SP, which works with the 207 CCGs [21]. Social prescribing pilots are usually done in collaboration with the H&B team and the Local Authority (LA). The first case which involved pharmacists with SP was Doncaster Social Prescribing [22]. This needs to become the norm across the UK but this requires a great deal of time investment and effort from pharmacists wishing to do a pilot in their locality, and several meetings with key stakeholders (CCG, HWB and LA) to allocate funding for SP. This is increasingly difficult for pharmacists working with chains of pharmacies due to the infrastructure of the organisation.

The new GPhC standards were released on May 12th, 2017, stating that we must act professionally at all times, including hours outside of the workplace [23]. This caused confusion within the sector, creating the perfect opportunity to introduce new ways of working with Social and Digital Prescribing. This complies with the following GPhC statement:

"All pharmacy professionals contribute to delivering and improving the health, safety and wellbeing of patients and the public. Professionalism and safe and effective practice are central to that role."

Community Pharmacy 2.0

On April 1st, 2005, the New Pharmacy Contract introduced MURs which was then followed by NMS on the October 1st, 2011 [24]. Both these advanced services better-enabled the pharmacists to increase their footprints within the community. This was further reinforced by the national flu vaccination which was started on September 16th 2015 [25]. For income stream, locally commissioned services can be contracted in collaboration with local stakeholders (CCGs, LAs & NHSE Teams). However, for pharmacists not involved with the Local Pharmaceutical Committee (LPC), it can be challenging to do a pilot with an associated budget.

Therefore, the solution I propose is a social and digital prescription. As a Medical NLP practitioner [26], I was able to do over ten consultations to improve the wellbeing of patients on antidepressants, with immediate success as I was empowering them in less than 5 minutes with the techniques I learned from the practitioner course. Equally, as I learnt more about nutrition, I was able to advise patients better on healthy eating and, as a result, patients felt more encouraged to go through dietary changes. For those who do the SCOPE course, it can provide a quality mark in your knowledge [27]. Furthermore, as I was explaining to patients about neuroplasticity regarding behavioural changes, they were more prepared to attempt lifestyle changes. I have also been recommending the use of BrainHQ to patients to maintain a healthier brain [28]. After attending the Nidotherapy conference, also being the first pharmacist to do so [29], the skillset developed then is one transferable to a community setting which would help patients gain empowerment. Those additional services will lead to an increased SROI (social return on investment). Another term to be introduced is the Patient Activation Measure (PAM) [30]. If all 44,000 community pharmacists provided similar services, this would greatly increase the self-efficacy of the UK population and solve the problems of the NHS.

References

[1]   DoH, www.gov.uk/government/uploads/system/uploads/ attachment_data/file/486941/letterpsnc. pdf

[2]   Chris Ford, www.npa.co.uk/2017/05/25/a-watershed-moment/

[3]   PSNC, psnc.org.uk/our-news/high-court-rules-pharmacy-funding-cut-was-not-unlawful/

[4]   NHS, www.england.nhs.uk/publication/nhs-five-year-forward-view/

[5]   NHS, www.england.nhs.uk/publication/next-steps-on-the-nhs-five-year-forward-view/

[6]   PSNC, psnc.org.uk/services-commissioning/locally-commissioned-services/healthy-living-pharmacies/

[7]   BBBC, www.bbbc.org.uk/the-early-days-of-the-bromley-by-bow-centre

[8]   SPN, www.westminster.ac.uk/news-and-events/news/2016/new-national-social-prescribingnetwork-addresses-nhs-healthcare-accessibility-issues

[9]   SPN, www.kingsfund.org.uk/events/social-prescribing

[10] Isobel White, researchbriefings.parliament.uk/ResearchBriefing/ Summary/SN05262

[11] CAB, www.citizensadvice.org.uk/about-us/how-citizens-advice-works/media/pressreleases/ almost-400million-a-year-spent-on-gps-doing-non-health-work/

[12] Neil Roberts, www.gponline.com/health-secretary-backs-gp-social-prescribing/article/1326032

[13] PV, pharmacyvoice.com/community-pharmacy/facts-and-figures/

[14] FOI, www.whatdotheyknow.com/request/how_many_registered_community_ph

[15] Statista, www.statista.com/statistics/318874/numbers-of-pharmacists-in-the-uk/

[16] RPS, www.ilovemypharmacist.co.uk/what-do-pharmacists-do/community-pharmacists/

[17] MHRA, www.gov.uk/government/news/is-your-app-a-medical-device-its-healthy-to-knowregulator-issues-updated-guidance

[18] RAENG, www.raeng.org.uk/publications/reports/health-apps-regulation-and-quality-control

[19] NHS, apps.beta.nhs.uk/

[20] NHS, www.england.nhs.uk/stps/

[21] NHS, www.nhscc.org/ccgs/

[22] SYHA, www.syha.co.uk/doncastersocialprescribing

[23] GPhC, www.pharmacyregulation.org/news/new-standards-pharmacy-professionals-come-effect

[24] BMA, https://www.bma.org.uk/advice/employment/gp-practices/serviceprovision/ prescribing/the-community-pharmacy/nhs-community-pharmacy-contractual-framework

[25] PSNC, psnc.org.uk/services-commissioning/advanced-services/flu-vaccination-service/

[26] Medical NLP, www.medicalnlp.com/

[27] WO, www.worldobesity.org/scope/

[28] Posit Science, www.brainhq.com/

[29] NIDUS-UK, nidotherapy.com

[30] King's Fund, www.kingsfund.org.uk/publications/supporting-people-manage-their-health

Movement Pharmacists
Needs To Unite

For this emerging field, we can call ourselves *"Movement Pharmacists"* as we are moving closer to patient-centred care, and we are enhancing the provision of pharmacy services via Social and Digital Rxs.

In September 2016, I founded *"Movement Pharmacy Association"* whose updated mission statement is:

"To maximise patient care and wellbeing using Social and Digital Prescribing with Neuroplasticity and Disruptive Technologies"

This is the promo video for MPA:

This is the promo video for "Dance for Seniors":

This is a table comparing the current model of pharmacy, which focus primarily in the supply of medicines, and the MP model, which was designed around the wellbeing aspect of the patient for prevention of ill health.

Current Pharmacy Model (Medicines Focused)	Movement Pharmacy Model (Wellbeing Focused)
Telehealth	Telewellbeing
GSL Stand	Wellbeing Stand
POM	Social & Digital Rxs
MUR	H&W Review
NMS	New Social & Digital Service
Annual Flu Vaccination	Annual Resilience Booster
Vitamins	Brain Exercises
Pharmacy Funding	Social Care & Public Health Funding
Health Worker	Wellbeing Worker
ACT	Wellbeing Technician

Current Pharmacy Model (Medicines Focused)	Movement Pharmacy Model (Wellbeing Focused)
Health Campaign	Social & Digital Campaign
Paid for Services	Paid for Health Outcomes
BP/Diabetes Check	Anxiety/Loneliness Check
Pharmaceutical Industry	Social & Digital Health Industry
Consultation Room	Meditation Room
Drug Tariff	Empowerment Tariff
NHS Health Check	Nidotherapy Assessment
British National Formulary (BNF)	Digital Health Formulary (DHF)
Health Leaflets	Bibliotherapy

Wellbeing Stands with Digital Medicines could include the following:

- Self-help/Meditation books;
- Memory Smell Products for dementia patients (e.g. grass, sea);
- Instructional videos for healthy living (exercises, nutrition and sleep);
- Audiobooks for personal development;
- Mobile Apps; or
- Augmented Reality (AR)/Virtual Reality (VR) headsets

| Accreditation Criteria for Movement Pharmacists ||
Areas	Providers
Physical Activity (e.g. Dance)	Dance for PD, EPE TBA, People Dancing
Behavioural Changes	The Society of Medical NLP
Mental Health	Meditation Instructors
Environment Analysis (e.g. Nidotherapy)	NIDUS-UK
Social Prescribing	TBA, Social Prescribing Network TBA, CPPE
Digital Prescribing	TBA, NHS Digital TBA, CPPE
Nutrition	SCOPE
Neuroplasticity	The Neuroscience Academy

Training fee for MP:

- £1,678 for Medical NLP License
- £204 for EPE
- £250 for SCOPE
- TBA for Social & Digital Prescribing Course
- TBA for Brain Science Coach course
- **Total of £2,132**

Intrinsic Value exponentially exceeds Monetary Value thanks to emotional contagion, priming and leadership skills acquired from Medical NLP courses.

This is an example on how government money could be spent to up-skill pharmacists in delivering advice for increasing the self-efficacy of the patient, which would alleviate current pressures on the NHS. This becomes even more important with the ageing population seen globally as a result of medical development and healthier living.

Pharmacoeconomics – Implementation Potential	
GP Pharmacist (GPP)	**Movement Pharmacist (MP)**
£112 million for 1,500 GPPs	£94 million for 44,000 MPs
28 patient interactions daily (PID)	40 PID
42,000 PID for 1,500 GPPs	1.8 million PID for 44,000 MPs
913,500 PI monthly (PIM)	39 million PIM
11 million PI yearly (PIY)	470 million PIY
110 million PI for ten years (PITY)	4.7 billion PITY

If you do a pilot of SP in your local area, you can use measures of the impact to justify the investment in the project.

Measure of Health Outcomes (before and after):

- The Wellbeing Star
- The Warwick-Edinburgh Mental Well-being Scale
- Work and Social Adjustment Scale (WSAS)
- Satisfaction Survey
- Qualitative experience, individual case studies and interviews on how social prescribing benefited their social lives and personal development

- Use of A&E, scheduled/unscheduled admission, cohort comparison with those receiving social prescribing interventions and a control group from another area with similar social-demographic measures

- Use of Read Codes by MPs in Health and Social Care IT systems across primary and secondary care (SCR)

- Formative Assessments

- EQ-5D Questionnaire

- Social Isolation Score developed by Elemental Software

This is how you could design planograms around prevention of ill health.

Pharmacy Planograms	Wellbeing Planograms
Cosmetics & Fragrance	Inner Beauty
Children Health	Parenting Skills
Digestive Health/Weight Management	Healthy Eating
Cough/Cold/Flu Health	Stress Coping Skills
Women Health	Women Empowerment
Pain Relief Treatment	Fitness
First Aid	First Aid Education
Vitamins	Brain Exercises

I did judo since the age of seven and I gained my black belt under the mentoring of Basil Dawkins at Moberly Judo Club in 2006. We are taught at a young age about eight virtues which I am passionate about and it helped me to develop the required grit. It enabled me to reach new heights both personally and professionally. These are the eight virtues:

- Self-control;
- Loyalty;
- Integrity;
- Courage;
- Compassion;
- Respect;
- Sincerity; and
- Honour

This is the model of MP which consists of three parts:

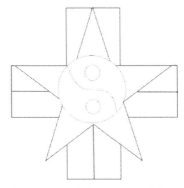

Movement Pharmacy Model

This is the first part "Yin Yang":

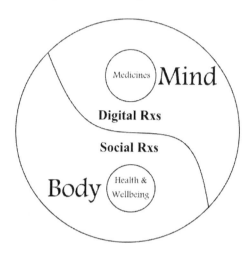

This is the second part "Pentacle" based on the *"The Five Giants of Society"* by William Beveridge in 1942, which laid the foundation for the National Health Service (NHS) in 1948.

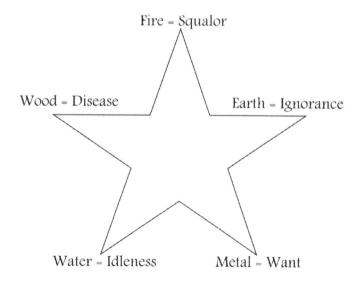

The key points are:

- Stress can be perceived as mental squalor if no coping strategies are developed;

- Health illiteracy, seen as ignorance, reduces the self-efficacy of the patient;

- People need to be educated on the different forms of wealth, and many of them only want money whist sacrificing their health and their family bond;

- Unemployment as idleness needs to be tackled by bringing a renewed sense of purpose through the creation of social enterprise and relevant opportunities like computer programming; and

- Medicines can treat disease, but we are not doing enough for prevention of ill health as value based care.

This is the third part – Cross – which embodies the eight virtues and four key areas of healthy living:

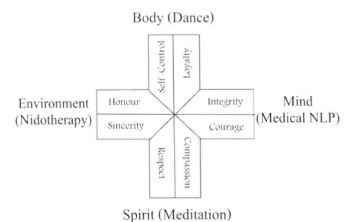

Body (Dance)

Self Control | Loyalty

Environment (Nidotherapy)

Honour | Integrity

Sincerity | Courage

Mind (Medical NLP)

Respect | Compassion

Spirit (Meditation)

Body can involve any physical activities like dance, mind would relate to your mindset on how to cope with stress, spirit is for your sense of purpose as in what makes you want to get up in the morning – do you have a fire in your belly to impact the life of others? – and the environment is stronger than your willpower so you need to analyse it for anything which can hold you back, including your circle of personal influences such as family, friends and work colleagues.

I did a keynote speech in Swindon about MPA in January 2017, this is the video:

Dance For Seniors (DFS)

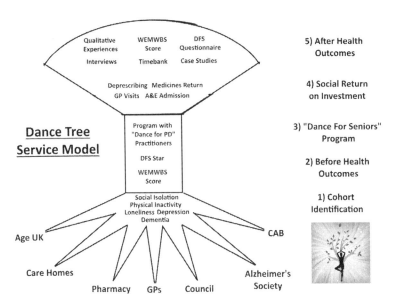

Dance Tree Service Model

- Qualitative Experiences
- WEMWBS Score
- DFS Questionnaire
- Interviews
- Timebank
- Case Studies

- Deprescribing
- Medicines Return
- GP Visits
- A&E Admission

- Program with "Dance for PD" Practitioners
- DFS Star
- WEMWBS Score

- Social Isolation
- Physical Inactivity
- Loneliness
- Depression
- Dementia

- Age UK
- Care Homes
- Pharmacy
- GPs
- Council
- Alzheimer's Society
- CAB

5) After Health Outcomes

4) Social Return on Investment

3) "Dance For Seniors" Program

2) Before Health Outcomes

1) Cohort Identification

DFS Star

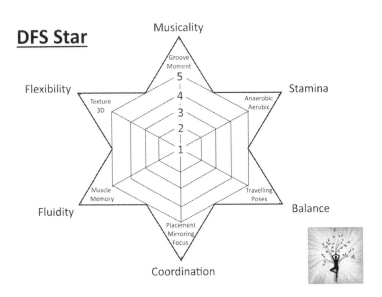

- Musicality
  - Groove Moment
- Flexibility
  - Texture 3D
- Stamina
  - Anaerobic Aerobic
- Fluidity
  - Muscle Memory
- Balance
  - Travelling Poses
- Coordination
  - Placement Mirroring Focus

Scale: 1 2 3 4 5

It is very important to be able to use a model in-order to engage the local stakeholders (LA, HWB and CCG) about your SP scheme. Using a questionnaire is also important to meet the criteria set out for a pilot. To measure improvement after each dance class, you can use a star to record it. This will provide a subjective view from the patient perspective. Additionally, using posters to engage the patients attending the pharmacy can be another helpful primer.

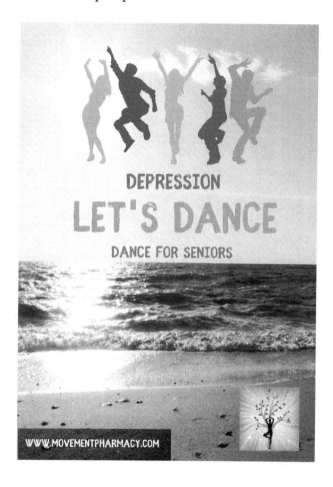

You can also work with your local GP surgery to promote SP with creative leaflets and packaging. This is an original version from another scheme in the UK (by Joe Magee with Dr Simon Opher OBE in Gloucestershire as "JoyN+").

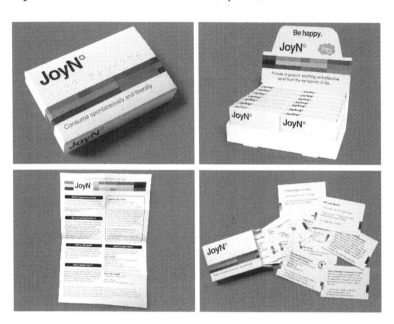

© Joe Magee

For example, the contents of the medicine box can be information about available SP schemes in the locality. I encourage you to contact Joe Magee to develop a tailored version, this is his website:

www.periphery.co.uk/joyn/

Digital Health Formulary (DHF)

Like the BNF, we could have one for digital apps as well as one for children like DHF for Children (DHFC).

The following was compiled from the NHS Beta App Store, MHRA website, personal recommendations, Dr Daniel Kraft TED videos & slides, Dr Bertalan Meskó book, attending the Health Plus Care Show in ExCel London in June 2017 and the Digital Health and Care Congress at the King's Fund in July 2017. It can be referred as DHF 2017 edition and it will eventually include AR/VR/MR therapy apps like Mimerse, MindCotine and VRPhysio from the consumer adaption of Extended Reality (XR) with headsets, smart glasses and smart contact lens.

DHF 2017

- AF – Kardia
- Asthma – MyAsthma
- Blood Pressure – Withings BP Monitor
- Bladder – Elaros
- Body Analysis – iHealth Scale
- Body Sounds – ThinkLabs digital stethoscope

- Cancer – OWise breast cancer
- Carotid – Mobisante probe
- COPD – myCOPD
- Dance – Desi Buck, Move it Or Lose it
- Dementia – Talking Point
- Dental – Brush DJ
- Diabetes – mumoActive, iBGStar, mySugr, Ayuda, mydiabetes
- Diagnosis – Scanadu
- Ear – CellScope
- Eye – EyeNetra, Welch Allyn iExaminer, Peek Acuity, Peek Contrast, Peek Red, Peek Colour
- Exercise – Salaso
- Food Allergy – FoodMaestro, FODMAP
- Healthy Living – Sugar Smart, NHS Smokefree, Be Food Smart, Easy Meals, Drinks Tracker, Couch to 5K, BMI Calculator, Smart Recipes, NHS Go, PHBChoices, Lincus
- Heart Rate – myheart
- Insomnia – Sleepio, Azumio Sleep Time
- Learning Disabilities – MyChoicePad, My Health Guide
- Lung – SpiroSmart Spirometer
- Medical Devices Techniques – Medhance
- Mental Health – Cove, Chill Panda, SilverCloud, Stress & Anxiety Companion, Ieso, Catch It, FearFighter, Headspace, Companion, Pacifica,

WorryTime, CBT-i Coach, Drinkaware, RR, Calm, PTSD Coach, Stay Alive,

- Feeling Good
- Motivation – Breakthrough with Tony Robbins
- Online Community – HealthUnlocked, Big White Wall
- Outcomes – LogPad
- Oxygen Saturation – Masimo iSO2
- Pregnancy – MyPregancy
- Prescription – Echo, Healthera
- Running – Run An Empire, Zombies Run!, my ASICS
- Sensor – Trichrome Healthcare
- Skin – Skin Scan, MySkinSelfie
- Social Prescribing – SPN (TBC)
- Surgery – Fit for surgery, Fit 4 Surgery
- Telehealth – Babylon, Push Doctor, Dr Now, VideoDoc
- Walking – Pokemon GO, Sweatcoin

DHFC 2017

- Alcohol – Start The Talk
- Asthma – Wizdy Pets
- Food Allergies – Wizdy Diner
- Vision – iSight Pro
- Walking – Pokemon GO

Interviews with Leading Authorities

I have done several interviews with world-class individuals from different areas of interest within Dance, Social Prescribing, Medical NLP, Digital Health, Meditation, Pharmacy, Neuroplasticity, NHS, Self-Efficacy and Healthy Living.

The purpose of these are to give you a framework to help you grasp the immense potential in preventing ill health with Social and Digital Prescribing. As a dancer myself, I have chosen Dance as one of the topics within Social Prescribing since this is the area in which I have the most experience. However, the benefits can also be applied in any social activities which emphasise social connectedness.

I have elected to leave it as transcript rather than paraphrasing, because everyone possesses a different mindset and they may interpret the information differently from the literal words of the transcript, as opposed to a paraphrased conversation. In addition, it maintains the authenticity of the message.

I invite you to empty your mind of everything you know about pharmacy, so that you can fully immerse yourself within the priceless content delivered by them. I highly recommended to read the book more than once after you have conducted further research for yourself on the topic.

These are a collection of interviews I have done since September 2016 and the book launch will be in January 2018. If you have any questions, please do not hesitate to contact me on:

arun.nadarasa@yahoo.co.uk

If you are inspired by the work laid out in this blue ocean, please do join the Movement Pharmacy Association to help spread the message within this book.

Interview with Amrish Shah from SuperMind

In community pharmacy, we only have a brief interaction with the patient when handing out medications to them. In 2005, the NHS (the UK's public health authority) introduced Medicines Use Review (MUR) which gives us 15 minutes with the patient to go through their medications, enabling brief lifestyle advice to be provided to the patient. This can only be done once a year as an enhanced service (it can also be done informally, but we will not get paid by the NHS).

Arun – Since non-useful habits occupy a larger area of the brain map as neuroplasticity took place, a brief conversation won't be enough for a change in more useful habits. How long should community pharmacists spend with the patient to enable the shift to occur?

Amrish – That is a very good question. Habit is a cause of re-wiring in the brain. There is a very scientific and cool new word called *"re-designing your brain"*. Re-wiring is basically about forming new habits and not holding onto the old 'bad' habits. It is not so easy to eliminate bad habits. One must have the awareness – it's still a hard part of the memory – but, like in childhood, you can have bad memories and have good memories. Later in life, you can overwrite the bad memories and control them forever if you know how to control your mind. So, neuroplasticity which you mentioned is so amazing and yet is only approximately 20 years old.

This is because neuroplasticity is all about defining the **final** frontier of science for mankind, which is the brain, with neuroscience applied: how to rewire the brain in the best way to create efficacy in neuronal cells. Different habits take different lengths of time to form. In general, the minimum period is around 20 days to change basic habits such as, for example, not taking a bath for a month; if you do not bath for a month you will not miss it. So, if you want to change into the habit of taking a bath regularly, it may you 20 days before you then get used to taking baths regularly. For habits which are much more deep-rooted, they take around 220 days. The general bracket is 20 days to 220 days for forming new habits, but with very conscious and diligent effort control coupled with a deep awareness of what you are doing.

The awareness of creating new habits and having a goal with definitive, specific objectives will determine how fast and how strong a new network will form and for how long it will stay. The tenacity, strengths, and difficulties will open up brand new pathways. For example, if you want to be a good hiker and you have never stepped foot outside of your comfort zone, you know that only travelling from your house to your workplace and other routine walks will not make you a hiker. If you then suddenly begin training to hike with a regime, you cannot achieve it in 20 days; it requires a lot more effort to rewire your brain to form that new ability, so it is between 20 and 220 days. It is also directly proportional to the effort and belief which you put into the task of learning to hike.

Arun – As a pharmacist, when I speak with the patient, I will need to inform them that a new installation of healthier habits could take between that timescale to become ingrained in their personalities. However, support will be given regularly to keep them on track and to ensure they reach their goal of forming the new habit.

Amrish – Brilliant, you are quite clearly doing a great job with explaining and intervening in patient care by going that all-important extra mile. Likewise, you have a great purpose with the distribution of knowledge of this amazing discovery known to mankind which is Neuroplasticity; you can apply a scientific concept for the formation of new habits. Arun, you can consult with me on a specific strategy if required – www.supermind. world. Make sure to tell your patients that it is going to take between 20 to 220 days, so that the patient is well-prepared to undergo the science of neuroplasticity. This way, you are not jumping the gun and your patient will not get disheartened with comments such as "*Nothing is really happening, Arun*" and "*What should I do?*" or "*This is not working!*" The moment they are aware of the scientific evidence of this new habit formation, they will be well-assured. Also, don't forget, motivation given to them meets a purpose when you know there are bound to be positive results.

The patient can adjust and dissect a little as they go along bringing that pertinent change, or healing their pain, wounds and ailments. We have learnt as neuroscience practitioners that it is very important to keep your patients in the correct light and in the right confidence. Sharing enough knowledge will make them realise the reality on how to move forward, rather than staying in the dark. The patient who is aware is also subject to mental instabilities, but usually they are quite able to accept the condition they are suffering from and that they want to cure themselves. This self-awareness makes the brain change, because it now matters; the brain changes swiftly when it matters to it. This happens along with medication and other scientific methods if prescribed. When you change into new habit formations and build new neuronal routes, the changes it can bring will form new patterns. The patients will get uplifted by rewards and results piece by piece, and they will work the way you want them to. The feeling of being rewarded at every little achievement kicks in the apt neurotransmitter in the brain, which enables motivation to work harder on the task.

Arun – It was found that motivation is key for adult plasticity to take place, there is the concept of 'gamification' to be applied to digital health to enable long-lasting changes, what are your thoughts on this topic?

Amrish – It is a brilliant idea, Arun. You are bang on. The big idea is that we are living in a technologically-savvy world. In a digital ecosystem with such huge geographical distances covered go along with adult communion. So, gamification is the key. We should be thanking technology and we should just not respect it but also apply it in a good way whenever the needs arise. Gamification is amazing and it is a huge part for fitness and wellbeing. There are new devices to measure and scale exercise, regulate blood pressure, cardio-vascular moderation, and measure sugar levels, etc. Everything now is technology-orientated.

Gamification will help new neuronal pathways. This is an amazing way to excite the patient, to keep the person onboard, always, and there is a very good neuroscience application to this and it is called the reward system. It is the release of dopamine and it triggers the area where the human brain knows it is going to be rewarded. It releases dopamine which is a feel-good neurotransmitter, it makes you feel stable, alive and kicking. Gamification will bring about the reward system and the moment it comes, that gratification will be a huge accelerator in getting into good mental and physical health. Gamification will also ensure brain health on the go and can be exploited in the upgrade and upkeep of varied cognitive skills.

Arun – BrainHQ developed Brain Exercises which can be accessed online, should similar products be offered in community pharmacies to speed up the onset of neuroplasticity? This was Dr Michael Merzenich's work (to slow down the risk of developing dementia as demonstrated from the ACTIVE study).

Amrish – Yes, he is my mentor and I have been using BrainHQ for one and a half years now. I hold Dr Merzenich in high regard, having read his books. I have been following his videos and I have interacted with a company called Posit Science of which he is the founder. He has designed, along with other scientists, several games and other content for BrainHQ. These artificial intelligence games helped me immensely. Since it has got various facets to it, it can be personalised to one person as per that person's requirements, or the objectives that need to be achieved. But, the most important part, in my experience and education, is neuroplasticity. It is a very important point which I am making, and you must take this with serious concern and significance. BrainHQ or any others brain games which are available online, subject to neuroscience research, scientific evidence-based and preferably designed and supervised by neuroscience practitioners will surge positive effects of neuroplasticity.

BrainHQ is the most authentic website. However, it should rather be practised under supervision because what happens is that, with my personal experience and with the experiences of others whom I have been training, the brain is getting re-wired in many ways throughout these video games. They are not just games for fun, but they are designed by neuroscientists and they do affect the neurology of the brain. So, one must be very careful, cautious and aware that one is going through this training and over a period, the brain is getting rewired and changes are being made.

Our reflex actions within the body are nothing but functions of the brain. You walk, you talk, you are listening which is what you are doing right now and absorbing, evaluating, paying attention, thinking, these are all brain functions. So, when you get rewired through video games like BrainHQ, the brain is changing its momentum, its function, its physiology and the body is still not being able to completely match up with it because the body is used to a certain pace and a certain momentum with a certain programming. Similarly, the mind and the memory are coping. So, it would be a mismatch and one could have kind of a knee-jerk reaction at times without even realising the brain has now changed, it has got faster, better and much more effective. That's why supervision is very important where brain science professionals like me, or any other neuroscience practitioner, are qualified to train others. That professional would be able to supervise a team of people who undergo this training, and once you have been guided and instructed from time to time, then the results that you see in your patients will be tremendous and will be very visible, and you will be scientifically quantified.

In short, what I am trying to say is that you should definitely think about and execute this plan if you have it in mind to train patients in BrainHQ, but you should undergo some kind of training to supervise them or have somebody who could supervise them appropriately.

Arun – So for me instead of saying come and do BrainHQ in the pharmacy, it is best for the pharmacist to work in partnership with a neuroscience expert, so that they can supervise let's say 20 patients at the same time or is it only on a 1-on-1 basis?

Amrish – It is 1-on-1, but the big idea is it's better to have somebody supervise in batch training, where you can have 5 to 20 patients, or whichever size is in demand, and have them come together. BrainHQ says that you should do it at least three times a week, which is about 90 minutes being 30 minutes a session or 5 sessions of 20 minutes. Personally, I recommend 100 minutes a week. The idea is that when it happens, we should have a batch training so that the services of a neuroscience practitioner or brain science expert is leveraged with a group of people rather than 1-on-1 training. If someone wants 1-on-1 and the neuroscience practitioner is available for that, then that's good enough too.

Arun – One of the ideas which I had in 2016 when I was reading his book Soft-wired was to identify patients whom may benefit from BrainHQ, and to work in partnership with the library to use their computers as many senior citizens don't have internet access. To work alongside the library around three times per week for 30 minutes, and now potentially a neuroscience practitioner could go with them to the library. This could be in a dedicated room to maintain confidentiality, but the addition of an expert does make sense because he can quantify the improvements like you said.

Amrish – Not just that, but to guide them correctly. Also you mentioned about dementia, which is a huge problem today in the world and sadly, it is going to grow; numbers are multiplying by the day. The world's aged population is increasing – more and more people are growing older. In the next few decades, it is going to be much more of a problem than it is now, which is going to bring about more cases of dementia or Alzheimer's with the largest rates today. I am very glad that you mentioned this. BrainHQ has proven that dementia cannot be completely cured, but the significance of damage can be reduced with BrainHQ. In fact, in Soft-wired, Dr Merzenich has mentioned about his mother in law suffering from it, and how she was cured by his expertise.

What you are doing right now about caring for the aged people and aiding people to organise supervised BrainHQ is an amazing idea. Neuroscientific evidence says that dementia cannot be completely cured by online video games, but games such as BrainHQ can bring down the percentage and seriousness of it, or even better it can prevent dementia which is absolutely evidence based. So, if you recommend neuroplasticity to older people or individuals advancing towards older age, in addition to supervised BrainHQ sessions, you are doing a great job because it is under the umbrella of Dementia or Alzheimer's which is the biggest rate of increase the world is facing, second only to depression of course. You should be very effective in bringing this change and helping these older people to never have to suffer dementia until the very end their lives. Applied neuroscience will help for long-term sustenance, but at the same time if somebody wants to continue this training for a year, or for many years, it will only help and keep their brains at the most effective performance levels.

Arun – Also, when you mentioned about the brain getting faster and stronger whilst the body is not able to keep up, this is why it is important to have a neuroscience practitioner. My idea was to combine BrainHQ with the library and dance classes, so that BrainHQ would make the brain faster and the dance classes would help make the body faster and stronger so that they can remember more dance moves.

Amrish – It is a terrific idea, any exercises are complementary to the brain's overall enhancement. Neuroscience research has clearly shown that those involving full body movement such as walking, running, cycling and of course dance, immediately benefit from the positive effects which the brain experience, and it stays healthy. Dance as a form of exercise combined with BrainHQ is a brilliant idea, and you are doing a great job by thinking about it. All you have got to do now is to execute it. I will try the same Arun, wish I was in your part of this beautiful world.

To get a neuroscientist's help is harder, as they will be fully focused on research and studying, so they will be too occupied. However, neuroscience experts or practitioners or brain science coaches will be apt for this kind of work. You can Google this to find a local practitioner and promote BrainHQ; I am sure you will find somebody and even a neurologist would be good enough for this.

Arun – Medical NLP involve the understanding of the brain process such as Deletion/Distortion/Generalisation (Meta Model), would Talking Therapy be enough to enable changes in the patient behaviours?

Amrish – Yes, any cognitive therapy is very important. The research has in fact stated that it is even better than pharmacology in certain ways or certain diagnosis. There is this amazing neuroscientist called Dr Norman Doidge, he has written books and inferred that the brain is the function of the mind and the mind is the function of the brain. So, what he is trying to say is that if you train your mind – which is what therapy is all about, which is what NLP is about or which is what any cognitive therapy is about – it will change the programming of the mind. The brain also changes, as does its physiology, and that is the most thrilling part, it is what neuroplasticity is all about.

Once the brain changes for the better, it changes the mind. The mind then further changes the structure of the brain towards better physiology and function. It is such a beautiful cycle – mind changing the brain and the brain changing the mind. The same thing continues like a circle; you are effectively getting to the right circle of Brain Health. NLP or any other therapy is also beautiful, it changes your thinking. The moment it changes your thinking, it starts affecting positively, constructively on the brain physiology, the moment the physiology of the brain changes, the structure changes, the wiring of the neurons changes, it again sets back in motion with a new order of thinking. A new order of thought process and a new order of habits like we have discussed earlier. These habits continue after a certain point of time, you automatically are rewired, and you have a new brain.

The mind dictates the neurons to fire together and the mind also – what Dr Merzenich said very importantly – is that the brain wants to find purpose in everything that it does. The moment the neurons find a purpose in what it should be doing – a meaning that this is the correct way – it starts firing together. The moment it fires together multiple times, it gets wired together. The moment it gets wired together, it remains that way and then it creates a new thought process. New pathways. New Destiny.

Arun – Everybody I speak to in regard to neuroplasticity do not know about it, so I start explaining it which reinforces my learning. I started to explain that concept to patients and they understand when I tell them it is important to think positively. For some patients, I recommend that they write a gratitude diary (Robin Sharma holy hour concept) to make change, and they find it very positive when I explain that is how the brain works and is wired to do so.

Amrish – Since you are doing such a great job, Dr Michael Merzenich framed those words with a great philosophy that "*all brains are work in progress*" meaning that when we are talking to people about neuroplasticity, about staying positive and maintaining a gratitude diary, you also are saying that your brain is a "*work in progress*". It is not complete, and it is not hard-wired so it is going to change. The gratitude, the positivity, the neuroplasticity can bring about the changes that you are always looking for.

Arun – Have you got any thoughts that community pharmacists should be aware of, to assist them in the health and wellbeing of patients?

Amrish – The most important things are what you have already said and are already practising, one word – neuroplasticity. I am also trained under Dr Sarah McKay, please Google her. She runs an academy called The Neuroscience Academy and she is a PhD graduate from the University of Oxford, a neuroscientist herself, she is running this academy with online training. Every six months, she opens for new students to join in. She has a brilliant syllabus and I have learned a lot from her. If you are interested, Arun, or anybody else in becoming a neuroscience coach or practitioner, please do join her academy, spread the word. What you are doing, what I am doing, what she is doing, what Dr Michael Merzenich is doing, what Dr Norman Doidge is doing, we are all in this together, on the same page, just at different levels. Our purpose should be finally to spread neuroplasticity and its benefits as far as possible.

Arun – Also if someone was to join The Neuroscience Academy led by your mentor, how long does the training takes to become a neuroscience practitioner?

Amrish – Brilliant question, Dr Sarah McKay has been a neuroscientist for the last 23 years. She has distilled all her knowledge and applied it to this academy. It works so brilliantly that if you can take it up, you can become a certified neuroscience coach within four to five months. You must take an exam and you must train with her, there are no time limitations, however. If you do not pass the first time, you can re-apply after six months and you automatically become a life-member of the academy. Similarly, if you have any questions, she is available to answer them.

Additionally, if anybody requires professional guidance, especially to overcome ailments, or wants to achieve any objective in any other part of their lives, then I am available for that. My email address is available on my LinkedIn page, as you know (supermindworld@gmail.com). My mission is to spread brain health around the world. My website is supermind.world,

Thank You Fraternity Neuroscience.

Interview with Linda Ray from Neuresource Group

Arun – Should we provide brain exercises to patients to reduce the risks of cognitive decline? Such as learning a second language, doing scrabble and cross-words as lifestyle advice to the patient who comes to our pharmacy, as many of them tend to be over sixties.

Linda – I think that pharmacists are ideally placed to be able to do more than what people think pharmacists do. This could be filling prescriptions and giving advice about how to take their medications. I think the idea that explaining the role to supporting pharmacists to give that sort of advice would be useful. We know from research literature that the benefits of training exercises and keeping an active mind do guard us from cognitive decline, I think that is something which would be very valuable as an open option to improve brain function.

I think people need to understand that mind training and keeping active are the only things which they need to do. It also allows you to learn more about how the brain functions. How can we learn something in a different way that might actually decrease some of stress we experience day-to-day, which will also contribute to the cognitive decline as well.

Arun – What's your opinion on using VR as a form of education for medical conditions during MURs?

Linda – I think that is a really good idea in terms of fun. When people experience something, they can imagine what it is like, they are more likely to remember something. We also know that people need to hear information at least three times before they have any possibility of remembering it. So, if we can provide it in a different a form other than written, or from a VR, that could be very useful. I think when we look at technologies we should do so from a perspective of how they may assist in developing new habits.

It could be during a new regime of medication; often people will forget important information and they may need cues and reminders that can support them to implement this new regime. The other thing also, is what are the ways in which we can support people to download information onto an app, so they can then access it on a just in time basis?

I undertook postgraduate studies in Neuroscience of Leadership, and I have been exploring how we can apply neuroscience concepts to leadership and the workplace. We know that you will be seeing patients in pharmacy who may have had a distressing diagnosis, so it elevates their stress levels, their cortisol goes up and that impacts negatively upon the hippocampus, the part of the brain which help us to encode information.

If people can be given information through various mediums, that enhances their capacity to be able to retain and hold on to that information. It can be through VR, with materials or using information and apps to go back to look at the information. I think that would be very useful indeed.

Arun – Amazon recently announced that they are intending to get involved within the pharmacy sector. Alexa is a device powered by AI. Anybody can touch it and ask a question and the device will respond back. It could be taught on different topics, and there was some discussion around its usage in care homes or patient home to help them with their medication.

When you mentioned the fact that people need to be told something three times in-order to remember it, Alexa could become a companion, especially for those who have memory issues like dementia to remind them about why they are taking their medicines. Would having a voice controlled device to help remind us about information be beneficial? Or would it be negative in terms of removing the social human-to-human connection.

Linda – I think that it sounds like a great idea and I can't help but relate it to my own experience, as I have two ageing parents. One of them has Alzheimers and my mother is seventy-six, so she has some memory problems. The point you are making about social connections we know as human beings, the brain is social, we are born to connect and that's an important human need. VR could be very useful, and I would hate to see that it may completely replace social connection and people interacting together.

They can't interact with a device, they can't ask questions that they don't understand. So, there should still be that interaction with another person to clarify things for them, I think that's important.

Arun – Regarding BrainHQ, both myself and my mother use it, speaking with Amrish who is a brain science coach, he recommended the supervision of a brain science coach who can monitor the progress of the participants as their cognitive function improvement may not match their current physical state. In your opinion, should we recommend seniors citizens to use BrainHQ and other alternative games?

Linda – At the moment, I am really liking a brain training program in Australia designed by an integrated neuroscientist Dr Evian Gordon. He developed a product called "My Brain Solutions", what I like about that particular program is the assessment which allows you to pinpoint cognitive functions that need to be improved. People may do brain training, but it may not be targeting the areas that they need to target. It might help with executive function, but it may not help with for example, recall or cognitive flexibility.

My Brain Solutions measures four key interdependent processes: emotion; thinking; feeling; and self-regulation. What Evian talks about and I think it's really important, that gets missed in some of the other brain training games, is that the assessment gives you a snapshot of how with your brain processes are in alignment. When that's not in alignment, that can cause problems for people.

This assessment allows you to look at the areas that are problematic from a cognitive capacity, and design a specific program to support you to develop those cognitive functions. One of the thing we've been experimenting here in the work that we do is including a brain assessment tool to support participants to understand their brain and how it drives their behaviour.

This is early days for us because we haven't included a brain training assessment tool in the past. So, we have just started to do the first debriefs of people and what's been really interesting is to see the improvements in their cognitive capacity and the alignment of those four different areas is improving.

The question for me is I think it's great to do brain training exercises, but I also think that people will actually need to have another component which helps them to understand how the brain functions. A classic example is, I don't know if you came across some of the work that Kelly McGonigal has referred to in thinking about stress, she's written a book called "The Upside of Stress". There is another bunch of research looking at mindset around stress where it significantly impacts us and affect us.

They talk about two different mindsets and I think about it as more of a continuum. There are people that have stress described as a debilitating mindset. They see stress as bad for them, stress is terrible and there are other people who see stress as good, as an enhancing mindset. It supports them to perform better, be at their best. What the research is showing is that your mindset about stress then significantly impacts on your physiology. If we say stress is something that can help us perform at our best, then we see less restriction of blood vessels when experiencing stress. What they've seen in people who see stress as bad for them, they get restricted which can lead to cardio-vascular issues in the future.

There is some research to suggest that cortisol is absorbed more quickly when we are stressing, as there are more cortisol receptors in the brain which guards against the negative impact of cortisol on the brain and body. It's alright for people to do mindfulness and all sorts of training you can do to help you keep calm, but we have to also be educating people to train their mindset about things, so that they can understand this is how it impacts your brain and body but you can do something about it by just changing your mindset about seeing stress in a different way.

It has a significant impact on health outcomes. There was a study done in the US which Kelly McGonigal refers to, and it shows people that saw stress as good for them and had experienced quite significant levels of stress in the past six months had a much lower chance of a bad outcome, like dying. In contrast, people that saw stress as bad for them and had significant high levels of stress in the past year, the figure is a 43 percent greater chance of dying.

The people who viewed stress as bad for them and had moderate level of stress had a greater chance of dying than the people who saw stress as good for them and had reported high level of stress in the previous six months. When you look at pharmacists, there is a real potential to be also sharing information like that, why couldn't you have a video that is shown while peoples are standing in line for ten minutes waiting for a prescription. It could be a ten-minute segment that people could have a look at, and might do some education to help them.

A perfect example would be "What's your mindset around stress?" and that would give people a chance to think differently and perhaps change their view of stress. The work by Alia Crum and Shawn Achor showed you can change mindset in three sessions of ten minutes' duration. If you could influence people's mindset to view stress as enhancing rather than stress as debilitating, I think that would be useful.

Arun – Yes, I did the Medical NLP course back in April 2017 which is different to mainstream NLP. I discussed with the founder about the possibility to improve the ability of patients to cope with stress, because we do flu vaccination to reduce the risk of developing it. Stress has been recognised as an epidemic by the WHO and we are not doing anything about it in community pharmacy. How about delivering a resiliency booster session as we don't want to remove stress, but only change their perception around it. This resonates with what you explained to me.

I personally feel if we are given the right training, we

could either do it personally, with the patient, or to have an experienced professional come into the pharmacy, like hearing tests with a company representative, to do three sessions of ten minutes' duration with the patient. With the NHS 5YFV and HLP accreditation, we are aiming to engage with the patient more closely as a health and wellbeing hub.

Linda – Yes, we are working on easy to digest information, as we know there is a stress epidemic right now. The issue is how do we challenge the way in which we view stress for it to be viewed as something that can help – it's a natural physiological response. The unfortunate part is that the old part of the brain still reacts to threats, whether they are physical or social in the same way. When faced with a social threat, such as someone telling you what to do or dismissing your idea, our body still reacts as if we are facing a sabre-toothed tiger. We have the same biological response. Stress can be viewed as helpful and that it is a normal physiological response that can actually go a long way to help me do very well in a situation.

Arun – If all community pharmacists in UK were equipped to provide advice on how to change mindset around stress, it will, without doubt, vastly improve the issues in the mental health sector.

Linda – Yes, mental health is a massive issue in Australia. We've seen a rise in the amount of young people presenting with mental health issues. My hunch is that some of this is related to digital technologies and the developments of social media, which is posing a great problem here in Australia, as well as the rest of the world.

Interview with Debs Taylor from Creative Minds

Arun – Your speech at the King's Fund was really inspiring, you took ownership of your wellbeing after attending the arts classes and I can relate to you using my background as a dancer. I am pretty sure if people are given this opportunity of an alternative to medicine, it can improve their overall H&W, just like you did. I am very confident that your story will inspire many people to follow suit. You could re-iterate your journey from the art class to where you are now.

Debs – I have had mental health issues from the age of eight where I had panic attacks. I have been in and out of services since then. Seven years ago, I took an overdose. I was told by a psychiatrist that I would always be medicated and that I will never be able to work again. I believed that psychiatrist because I had been medically retired from my last job and I have been on benefits for fourteen and half years. So, I had no reason to believe anything else. From my overdose, I was referred to the crisis team who referred me to see a psychologist and it was while I was sat in the waiting room, I saw a leaflet "Arts for Wellbeing" by Creative Minds.

I had never done arts before, but I picked the leaflet up and I rung the number where they said to come along to a taster session. I went along, and I really enjoyed it. In the six years that I have been doing it, I sold one hundred and fifteen paintings, I had an exhibition at Canary Wharf in London, I am no longer on the twenty-one tablets a day that I was at the time I took the overdose. I am no longer a service user. I have been out of services for nineteen months now.

I am working for the first time in fourteen and a half years, something which I never expected to be doing. I do talks about my journey all over the country. Initially, I started to do them to give service users some hope because I felt that wasn't in the system. I felt that telling people that I will always be medicated, and I will never work again didn't inspire me whatsoever. So, I wanted people to know that things can be better than what you are told. That these experts do not always have the answers we are looking for. Maybe sometimes we have the answers within ourselves? Maybe we need to work together to find the right solutions to some of our problems and illnesses.

The professionals started listening and asking me to do talks at their events, which I do. I talk all over the country now about my journey, about mental health, anti-stigma, suicide awareness and suicide prevention. It is more about awareness for people and for them to realise that there are better options out there. We are not just defined by the illness and we know who we are. Also, to relay to the professional that even though they have letters and numbers after their names, they are not necessarily an expert in each person's individual condition. This is because nobody knows that condition better than the person who lives with it twenty-four seven, and we need to work as a team to find more successful and productive solutions.

I still have the illness, they haven't magically vanished, they are still with me, I still live with them every day, but I have ways and means of managing and coping with it now. I spent two years doing the art classes and then I got my own studio, I have just moved to a new studio and I do arts from home as well. It's still a fundamental part of my journey. I still use it as my wellbeing tool to deal with the pressures and struggles of everyday life as well as maintaining my illnesses.

There is so many different chapters and areas that I never thought would be possible (for an invisible service user like me) and I would have never dreamt were possible. This is about people trying different things; it's worth having a go because you have got nothing to lose. I was put on a nineteen-month waiting list; the art class had no waiting list. If it does not work, you have not lost anything by trying it.

Arun – At the King's Fund event, there was another person who gave a speech, his name is Mr Trevor Fossey. He is an example of an empowered patient. Essentially, he was in a similar situation as you for a different medical condition, he had a stroke. He was explaining in his speech that once he took ownership of the data available for him, he was able to make better lifestyle decisions and he got reduced from six medicines to only two as well as reversing his diabetes.

Now, he gives speeches as part of "Patient Group Forum" where he is actually a champion in trying to have more patients become empowered. For them to receive more information about their medication, and about their wellbeing. In your situation, you could be described as an empowered patient because you took ownership of your H&W rather than giving the responsibility to somebody else. There is this movement in America about empowered patients and there is a website available to gather those patients to follow the same philosophy.

You are one hundred percent right. At the end of the day, we only have a snapshot of your health parameters but the patients are the expert of their own health and body. They will have a better understanding on what work and what doesn't. You also mentioned the fact that rather than just taking medicines, the condition is still there but you were able to cope with it better through arts. Therefore, I am writing this book on SP for community pharmacists to be better informed in offering it alongside medical advice.

Recently, I came across an SP scheme in Swindon called "Live Well Referral" under the public health section on PharmaOutcomes. This is how the information is relayed from the pharmacy to the organisation that can provide remuneration for the service provision and to keep an audit for quality assurance. I was able to use it twice for socially referring the patient to a community navigator also known as link worker. Both patients were very pleased, and I could see that from their facial expression. Once I explained to them that it was free and that they take ownership of what they would like to do, I was enabling them to become empowered for their wellbeing. I really hope that community pharmacists will share the same level of enthusiasm as I do for SP. Some GPs are offering it already, but community pharmacies are behind due to lack of awareness.

My personal journey with SP came by luck. In September 2016, I was at the RPS Annual Conference and I made the decision that I wanted somehow to combine pharmacy and dance. This is when I came across the term SP for the first time during my research and writing a book is the best medium for raising its awareness amongst my peers.

I founded "Movement Pharmacy Association" as a result, for moving the patient from one state to another which could be through more physical activity, more mental wellbeing and healthier diet. Your personal journey is extremely inspiring.

Especially with the fact that you are now able to inspire many other people by doing public speaking.

Debs – Yes SP is out there in the physical sector, it is not as active as it can be, but it is more acceptable. Whereas in the mental health sector, people think you cannot make decisions for yourself, you are not able to do things for yourself. I think you should give people a chance, let them have a go, let them see if they can do things for themselves. We get some really good results from it. People are managing their condition, people are taking ownership for themselves, living their lives they never thought was possible.

Arun – Yes, almost giving them more options rather than being medicine-focused. I completely agree with you.

Debs –To let patients take ownership of themselves. From a patient perspective, I have always been treated like a number, I have been a statistic in the system, I never had an identity, I never had that ownership because everybody has always told me how to behave and what I should do. Allowing people to become more than just their condition and their patient number, giving them their identity, giving hope meaning and purpose in life, surely that's what everybody should strive for not only for themselves but for others.

If that's all you've ever known, that's all you do. You are not aware that there is anything different out there. Once you are aware, then the world is your oyster. I see what I do as two parts, I want to inspire services users (patients) to think like that, that they can achieve more than what they would like, or are led to believe they can achieve. Secondly for the professional, they need to realise that just because we've got mental health conditions, it doesn't mean that we can't make decisions about ourselves. We need to work as a team to find the right solution for each person. We need to offer as many choices and options as we possibly can to enable people to manage better.

The more we empower people to start making decisions about themselves, the more likely we are to start building confidence to be able to do everyday things and make the right rational decision. If they can come off medications as well, then that's fantastic. I know my journey has been long, I still wonder *"Oh, that's happened to me"* and I am still in awe and amazement from having been in the system for forty years that this part of my journey happened in such short space of time. It's just wow, why didn't I find this out before. I can't look back and say *"Well, I should have found this twenty years ago"* because I may not have been ready then. It enabled me to find myself, I found my own solution. The right time and place can be crucial to recovery, but I think people should always be encouraged to keep trying new (and old) things in the hope that this time it might work out.

Arun – I am a strong believer that everything happens for a reason, there is this quote that goes *"When the student is ready, the master appears"*. It means that when you are ready to learn, that's when the pathway to your goal opens. Essentially, SP at every point of access within the NHS would empower people from any age group and of any medical condition, and would have such a tremendous benefit to both the patient and NHS overall. This is because when a patient gets a minor ailment, they can either go to the pharmacy or to a doctor. If it's really bad, they may go to A&E.

The only time where the expectations can be managed through wellbeing as in SP are currently done at GP surgeries. However, with the Social Prescribing Network (SPN) and the support of STPs, the whole phenomenon for SP becomes more mainstream. So, people become more aware of it and as a result, they can make better lifestyle decisions. By knowing more, they become empowered.

When I was speaking with Trevor, he mentioned about having the conversation recorded during consultation with the patient. This enables the patient to remember the content even after three or four weeks afterwards. That recording can be passed to their loved ones, enabling a better delivery of care. I am also working on VR as a medium of education where the topic on healthy living can be covered and made fun through gamification for young people.

Debs – Regarding spray arts, there is this device which connects to your computer and it projects a picture in your wall, you are told when to spray paint and it squirts at the right time as you move your hand along. You need a very steady hand to get it nice and straight and exactly the way you want it to be. I found it marvellous on how technologies can allow you to do that even if you are not really an artist. You can do it on murals and walls. It's just another option if you do not have the confidence to put pencil (or paintbrushes) to paper.

Arun – It's still early stage but VR can also be used to show social activities that are available in the locality to the patient. This will enable them to make a better-informed decision on whether they like it or not, by changing their initial perception with 180 or 360 videos as demo tour. It can be dance class, yoga class, art class or even gardening within the pharmacy premises in the consultation room. They can become immersed from the taster session where VR experiences can be the substitute for words. This enables the patient to become empowered through SP. What's your opinion?

Debs – It sounds incredible. I don't know why I picked up that leaflet on that day at that time, but I did, and it changed my life. My girls used to ridicule my arts. If you can give somebody a taster on what you got to offer, then the more likely they will try it out, then maybe decide to take it up. If they don't like dancing, they could do gardening so they would have more options rather than having to go a session and feel embarrassed that they were not as good as others. I think it's an amazing idea.

Arun – Yes, I was inspired from VR being used in paediatric hospitals in Poland where the founder goes to the cancer ward, and the patient must remain there for a prolonged time period due to the nature of the treatment. The children are shown VR videos as distraction therapy to allow them to momentarily escape from their current environment. The experiences include flying, riding a horse, climbing mountains, being in a forest and to be in the sea. They did a similar thing in Australia with adults who have cancer to help them go through the treatment.

In 2016, Mimerse – a VR company – offered pain relief through VR in Sweden's largest chain of pharmacies. The real-estate sector also uses VR to show clients what houses they have in their portfolio, without having to physically go the house to save time and money. This is how I was able to connect the dots on VR's potential as SP tasters in community pharmacy.

Debs – I think the NHS are trying to embrace SP. I would like to see everybody offered SP as well as traditional treatments because I know we can't magically make people feel better with only SP. Sometimes, you must provide the clinical part as well.

However, people should have the option. We are all experts of our own body. We need to embrace it and focus on moving forwards. SP transformed my life and its effective, why wouldn't we want to access something that has that much power? After all you have not lost anything by trying.

Interview with Trevor Fossey from Coalition for Collaborative Care

Arun – Your speech at the King's Fund was very inspiring. You are a role model on how patients should be empowered.

Trevor – Yes, from my background, I used to be with DHL supply chain as a global quality manager. So, quality and ensuring that all stakeholders were engaged in projects was very important. Then I thought there was never a way that I could get involved as a stakeholder in my own health, because I did not have digital access to my own health record. Access to information enables empowerment which is what I used to engage all stakeholders when I installed a quality management program globally within DHL, that was rolled out to circa. 2000 sites throughout 56 countries. All colleagues were engaged within that in lots of different languages. But, I realised that this element was missing from the NHS to some extent, I did not feel empowered to be engaged actively in my own health. I felt that 'treatment' for my ill health was something being done to me (the patient) without necessarily involving, or empowering, me.

I felt that people should be empowered. I got involved at that stage and I found that the DH Power of Information Power of Information initiative had been published in 2013. I asked my GP when I am likely to get that, to get engaged and he didn't know about it. My GP, however, was positive and said that I could join the Patient Participation Group (PPG) and ensure that the issue was on the agenda.

Aside from lots of reasons given by the GP Practice initially as to why access to records was not feasible, the practice agreed to give digital access to some patients, on a trial basis, in January 2014. That was the background of my initial involvement – because of the experience I had in my working role prior to retirement I had a vision of how things could be changed if patients were empowered. So, since January 2014, I have had digital access to my records and I have used the information to improve my own health. I was asked to get to involved at the King's Fund because Dr Brian Fisher knew my story as one of the members of the coalition of collaborative care and to encourage people, particularly those with long term illnesses, to be patient-centred, listen and treat the patient, not the illness.

In March 2017, I also did a talk in Southampton to persons who are living with diabetes – I was asked to go down for NHS England. The whole basis of that story was that access to your own record is important, and that it could be used to promote more engagement. The message given was that others don't have to follow specifically what I have done, but feel empowered to adapt it to their own individual needs. I personally decided that I needed a plan to achieve it. I had been told that I should do more exercises, but a stroke had left me with a mobility disability which makes exercise difficult. So that was out of the window, they weren't even thinking about that, not giving patient-centred advice. The other thing I was told was that I should not weigh myself every day as it would be demotivating.

Having worked in a commercial organisation, I did want to weigh myself every day, I wanted to note the changes. There, we are looking at things like peaking performance almost on an hourly basis for different people. It's got to be set around the individual I think; it needs be patient centred for the individual, but the advice that I received I felt was paternalistic, not considering the individual. The individual needs to be engaged; when I had a stroke, clinicians said *"Don't do this"*, I didn't want to go to any groups, I wanted to be involved myself. I think having a template for people, with IT to some extent, where you get algorithms with all different things that suit the individual, would be a more patient-centred approach. I am passionate about that and I welcome the opportunity to tell people the story.

Arun – Definitely, if most people follow what you did, their H&W will go to a very high level. Essentially, you have been pro-active in taking care of your H&W and as a result, you have been able to reverse your diabetes and only take two medicines now.

Trevor – Yes, one of them is aspirin because I had two strokes in the past. There is a risk of further stroke. To be honest, I don't take them every day, I haven't ordered it for the past three months but I will make sure to measure my blood pressure again. I will get a blood test and probably within the following hour, I will get the results to come through, and I can compare them myself, I can be 'engaged' with my own health in this way.

I made a comparison to my financial side, like I can get to my bank account 24/7 and I am in control of it. With your health, you should feel similarly engaged. The one thing I would say is you know, I've thought it was just the sort of culture within the

NHS and wellbeing generally and pharmacists to some extent as well as other clinicians that they took the view *"Hey, you don't really know about your health"*, and *"you can't be trusted with your own health"* I think that if people are made to believe those statements, they will behave in a manner that is expected of them.

I initially thought it was this paternalistic view that was stopping people becoming engaged in their own health, but I have since identified from speaking with lots of patients that they also need a cultural change as well because they have 'accepted' the paternalistic view that they don't know about their own health and they don't deserve to know what's happening, so they just leave it to the professionals instead of expecting to get involved in their own wellbeing.

We need to change the culture, to persuade people that there are some benefits in getting involved and engaged. One thing I do mention in some talks is my diabetes. One person in Southampton said that *"You should just trust doctors and you shouldn't get involved in your own health"* and I responded, saying *"I see a GP or a pharmacist once a year to be prescribed the medication and I see them for about an hour a year; but I live with the condition for 8000 hours a year, so who is the expert in my own condition?"*. If you put it like that, we patients are experts and if we did unlock that potential, it could achieve a lot. That's my belief anyway.

Arun – Your view is inspiring. There is also a person in America who did a similar thing with cancer. Luckily, his doctor was supportive to help him receive more information through technologies, and became empowered as a result. He founded a website to gather more people like him to empower patients. You are completely right, doctors probably only see a patient for 10 minutes per consultation. Whereas, the pharmacist sees the patient several times a year during MURs, medicine collections and the patients are the experts of their own body.

Through the increased use of wearable trackers, people will become more familiar with some of their health parameters. Dr Meskó, also known as The Medical Futurist, takes his health parameters on a daily basis, if he notices something is not right, he will then bring those results to his GP. Almost everybody owns a smartphone, Apple and Google are trying to include more health trackers in their watches. Patient will be able to bring more than one result, not a snapshot, ranging from one week to a month, to bring it to the attention of the doctor or the pharmacist.

We will be able to advise them better when looking at the spikes or unusual results in one of their parameters. This can help us adjust their medication regimen as well as wellbeing advice. Now, pharmacists are only focused on medicines. With my book, I will be aiming to raise the awareness of the wellbeing aspect through patient empowerment like yourself.

Trevor – I think pharmacists need to recognise that people are interested in their own health, but they feel that they need permission to be engaged. Like any projects in which I have been previously involved, it is very important that you engage the stakeholder; the patient is a major stakeholder in their own personal health. They're often given the impression that how things are decided for them without them. If we say *"Yes, it's down to you"*, you can give them the feeling that they got the power to get involved.

I know with my own situation when I was actively trying to do something last year, I was monitoring my sleep with a band. I could see what was happening and I could see what I've felt. I also monitored my blood results where I felt empowered. Actually, I went for a blood test at the hospital and I had an email with the results within three hours even before the doctor received the results. I felt this was empowerment and engagement which means I am getting involved.

With blood test results I don't have to phone the GP and wait for a week. I can see the results straight away, I can go to my computer. The empowerment is the main thing as I can remind myself of what happened, I can look back at notes from GP appointments that I have had in the past and review comments and what was said at the time or even reminders, and check whether I am doing what was suggested. I don't have to remember as you realise, people don't remember everything that was said to them particularly in a stressful situation.

For example, the pharmacist saying something should be noted on the records, maybe the GP health record. The pharmacist conversation should be noted there so that the person, in their own time, can have a look at that, and remind themselves. In particular, elderly people may not have access or feel comfortable with getting it on the network, they can go and see their son or daughter who can confirm what the pharmacist said about their pills. At the end of the day, it's their decision whether to share it but at least they can get comfort and an explanation from people they know well.

Arun – Yes, pharmacists have access to SCR but it's read only and we cannot add entries. However, NHS Digital are working toward enabling this feature. This is so that when doctors have access to this, they can see any key points raised by the pharmacist that may benefit patient care and wellbeing.

Trevor – This could be helpful for you guys as well. I know that there's been a patient who said to me recently that the pharmacy they've been into, said to them they would like a review of their medications, he said *"I already had one a couple of weeks ago with another pharmacist, why do I need to do it again?"*. You should have the information yourself, you should be able to see what was said last time and they should be able to come back to the patient, sit them, start the computer and take it onboard.

How many times have you been to a meeting where you are suddenly called in, like when you ask a patient to come in. Let's say that you have been to the bank and somebody called you in for a ten minute meeting, explained something to you and then two weeks later, will you remember in detail all that was said? So why are all these things said to the patient, with the facility to allow the patient to review the detail in their own time?

Arun – That's a good point. One of the thing I am working on is education through VR. There is lots of evidence that VR is an excellent platform for education as people become immersed within the medium. It will cover different medical conditions which can be accessed through the internet. It can include how to use their inhalers where they can refer to it later. It is more entertaining and easier to remember (the principle of gamification).

Trevor – Certainly, if they had a link to your initial conversation, if they are a child or an older person, they could go back and say *"I was shown this. This is what the pharmacist said to me and there is a link within that"*. They click in the link and they share the information with their loved ones. You can support them in using it properly.

Arun – Potentially, they could record the conversation in their smartphone for example, so that they can listen to it afterwards. That's a good point. I think that's a brilliant idea.

Trevor – I voice my views quite a lot, I share information as I did with the presentation. When I was coming to retirement, I had a problem what the GP said, *"You are depressed"*, I needed to know what he meant by that, and researched information when I got home and read his comments on my health record. As a result, without any medications, I was able to resolve the issue that and it was probably the trigger for me to get involved a bit more with the NHS.

A lot of benefits can come out of it, that's why I believe in SP. The individuals are encouraged to decide for themselves how they would like to get involved. They may want to join something like gardening or community projects. I like using my experience from the organisational world, which is about quality and running projects, for making a difference. Let's change the culture.

When I was working with an organisation, I realised that to engage stakeholders, I needed to empower them – and that would help me to change things and make a difference. Prior to getting involved with the Power of Information Initiative, I wasn't making a difference, I wasn't able to influence things. That's what turned me on, helping people develop and change culture, that's what I wanted to do. We need to recognise that everybody is different and individual, you don't try to help somebody else to be something like that, you need to find out what's within you to become a culture of engagement in your own health.

I am sure you don't use your bank account access like I do, I am sure everybody in the room does 'their own thing', so why should it not similarly be available in the health side of things where you need to be more involved? Effectively, you are in control of your own health and wellbeing – or should be – and I think that a culture change will help, and that it would encourage patients with their 'engagement' and wellbeing.

There is now software than can easily convert audio into written words if people want to. Also, for those who have some learning disabilities, so you must think about the different mediums used.

Interview with Dan Hopewell from Bromley-By-Bow Centre

Arun – I am aware you did some work with pharmacists already with SP, and you mentioned the fact that you will be attempting to look at it again. I would like to know how is it coming along?

Dan – I will have to check on how it is developing as I am not sure myself, as it is not me personally who is taking that piece of work forward, so I can certainly connect on what happened with the development on SP and the local pharmacies. I know there are many schemes in the country that are using pharmacies as part of their work. I think it's true to say that because the role of pharmacies is changing and there is an appropriateness for pharmacists to socially prescribe. I can come back to you and let you know, I can find out from our team here how those discussions are going with the pharmacists.

Arun – In terms of mobile applications being involved with SP, I am aware there are quite a few presentations mentioning how having it could facilitate the process of SP. My question is do you see that becoming more mainstream because almost every single citizen in UK owns a smartphone, and ideally having a mobile app to enable them to become more involved with their care. Do you see it becoming available within the next few years called "Social Prescribing Network" (SPN) where any patients could use it to get in touch with their social prescribing scheme within their locality, almost like Uber.

Dan – Yes, I am sure that will come. I think that's very interesting, I think what's being talked there of the idea. Now, I guess most SP starts with a referral from a HCP who is the person who see the patient and identify that need in the patient and then make the referral to the link worker. At that point, he or she contacts the patient and may signpost the patient to a service if they feel the patient have the level of motivation, self-efficacy and capacity to access whatever they need on their own without further assistance. They will signpost them but if they feel the patient would benefit from seeing the link worker, they will arrange it.

Most SP schemes will have a facility where the patient can come and see the link worker and at that point, they will more often go in from a ten minutes consultation with a HCP to maybe an hour with a link worker. So, you can have a much more in-depth discussion, and it may be at a slower pace consultation with the patient, it supports the patient in talking about their lives and what's important to them, and helping their patient to find out what will help them.

Now, the concept of an app or some sort of digital facility is interesting, and it potentially goes to many things. So, one might be once the patient has been socially prescribed, they might then contact their link worker using an app and they could stay in touch with their link worker through a messenger service. The other thing I guess that you are sort of alluding to is, of course, eventually once an SP scheme will have this sort of facility, patients can self-refer to the link worker without having first to see a medical professional.

I guess what you are saying is that, or what's behind your question is, really the question of will we get to the stage where patients or people in our community can self-refer to the link worker using a digital tool, and I think the answer will probably be yes. We will eventually get to this situation with the number of SP schemes. As I said, patients don't need first to see the doctor to see the link worker, they can self-refer and indeed some of our SP schemes are already experimenting with the idea of patients being able to self-refer to the link worker without having first seen the doctor.

I guess then we will need to probably think about all sorts of ways in which patients might be supported through digital technologies, so once the patient might be able to contact the link worker in their local area digitally. Another might be the patient keeping touch through the link worker digitally, whereas the other may be patients being able to connect with each other. So, you can imagine if you have a whole lot of patients who got a similar health condition, they might be able to form a group where together they support each other.

Arun – This reminds me of the company HealthUnlocked, which is the equivalent of Facebook but with people who share the same health conditions. They get to support each other, and it was shown from the data gathered that the patient wellbeing and health has improved by up to 30 percent. Essentially, it has been validated.

Dan – In times gone past, we all used to call this "self-care" and "self-management". These are two common terms which have been used in health for a long time. About teaching patients how to manage their health themselves, particularly if they have a LTC. One of the ways you could do self-care and self-management is to get patients to work together with each other. So, they support each other as a group. I guess that digital technologies will allow patients to be able to link up with each other using it.

I am sure there will be lots of ways in which digital technologies start to support both SP, but also some of the thing that come from SP. I mean, another thing is a lot of people who are socially prescribed are because they are socially isolated, for example. So, social isolation is a big issue in our community and of course, one can certainly see very easily the opportunity that digital technologies have for helping to reduce social isolation. I think that your question is correct because there will be lots of ways in which digital technologies help to support SP and the things people get prescribed.

Arun – I remember from attending the open day at BBBC in February 2017 that the way SP is funded is through private investors and some money from the CCGs and potentially HWBs including LAs. From the SP conference back on the 18th May 2017, there was a mention of that there could be a funding stream allocated for SP available from 2018. In your opinion, where should the money come from? Should it be directly from the NHS? Should it be funded directly by the UK citizens? Shall we involve private sector companies such as Virgin Care to get actual funding for the SP scheme nationally in your opinion?

Dan – Just to clarify, yes, now, SP funding is mainly coming from statutory sources. The private investors are invested in something called the "Social Impact Bond" which is one particular scheme in Newcastle. That, I think, is probably the only one that has private investment. Do you know how they work?

Arun – No, I never heard of it.

Dan – Social Impact Bond is the idea that you get investors to invest in something to get something started, but eventually somebody else will pay for the output and provide the longer-term incomes, based on what you achieve. So in the case of Newcastle SP scheme, it's a seven year programme and they got funding for the first couple of years from a social impact bond which is a social investment fund that is paid back, if the agreed outputs are achieved.

The money is to get the program started and get it running for the first couple of years. But, later, the investors are paid back by another funder based on the achievement of the outcomes. So, the question then is how do they pay the investors back. The way they pay the investors back is that they have agreed with the health authority in Newcastle that if they achieve certain outcomes with the patients, they will get paid for those outcomes.

So, the outcomes are improvements in the people health and wellbeing scores on a H&W scale. Basically, the whole premise of the funding is if you improve the H&W, they will use the health system less and if you can improve it by a certain level, you can assume a certain level of reduction in the healthcare costs for those people. So, the scheme in Newcastle, it has to show that the hundreds or thousands of people it works with what was their H&W score was at the beginning and what it was at six monthly intervals for twenty-four months. If it can prove or show that it increased their patients' H&W, the health authority in Newcastle then assume that those hundreds or thousands of people will have reduced their health expenditure cost because their H&W has increased.

Therefore, that would allow the health authority in Newcastle to pay the SP scheme a certain amount of money for each patient for whom they have improved their wellbeing, and the amount of money is less than the reductions in healthcare costs are. The health authority benefits because their healthcare expenditure has been reduced and is expected to reduce, and the SP scheme earns its income because it can show that it increased the H&W of the patient who has been socially prescribed. That money from the health authority pays back the investors for the money they borrowed to get the scheme running in the first couple of years.

It then also provides an ongoing funding for the scheme for the remaining years of the program. So that is what a private investor model is, but the investment is only just to start the thing for the first couple of years. In terms of who should pay for SP, I think we believe that the state should pay SP. Of course, the state in Britain has lots of different pots of money and I think it's interesting. Up until now, most SP schemes have been funded by a variety of sources. But, in terms of state money, most of that money has been to do with health or social care. What I think is interesting to think about maybe for the future is that lots of parts of the state benefit from SP. It's not just the health sector, you could argue that if you can improve somebody's life, there would be lots of part of the state who will benefit from that improvement.

Let's just look at a very simple example. If you get somebody who has been unemployed for a long time and they have a LTC, they lost their employment and then you socially prescribe them to the scheme and it help them work on their LTC and helps them to think about maybe getting some new skills, inggetting another job and then eventually, they will join some courses, get some training, get some new skills and then they get the job.

You can start to see lots of financial benefits to the various parts of the state through that one person. Their health may improve because they have been given support around their health condition, you may start to get a reduction how frequently they go to the doctor, for example, because of this improvement. They may also have less medications, so they become less expensive in terms of the drugs they need. You may think whether they get a job, they stop receiving unemployment benefits or health-related sickness benefits, and they may start paying taxes as a citizen and an employee now earning a salary.

You start to think about, how through SP, that one individual has improved their health, they stopped claiming social benefits, they start paying taxes. You may say that their children are more likely to do well at school because their parents are now working and have become a role model and example for their children.

You can start to think of a whole series of positive benefits for that person and their social behaviour. They may also be less likely to be in debt as they are working, so have less problems. All sorts of situations may improve through that person. It may have all started around SP. Therefore, you may argue that it's not just the health system that should be paying SP, it's quite plausible to argue that entire parts of the state system and different states pot of money may all contribute to the funding of SP.

Presently, SP funding is largely limited to the health world. I think, hopefully, we will get to a point where we will have a much broader understanding of where the benefits accrue from SP. Therefore, we will have a much broader understanding of who may fund and finance SP.

Arun – My question is about Universal Basic Income (UBI). From what I remember, I was watching a TED video and there was an article released in 2016 saying that by having a UBI, it is going is to enable the citizens to go from a scarcity mindset to an abundance one. Therefore, they are going to be more empowered to take more healthy decisions because they don't have to focus all the time about how to raise money. So, by not having any financial stress, it may improve their H&W so where do you see UBI complementing SP essentially. For instance, you could start with a small pilot where all the citizens in one city don't have any benefits, they all get UBI regardless they are employed or not. There were few test cases in America.

Dan – I know there has been case in Scandinavia maybe or in Northern Europe. I think there are some places with small scale experiments with UBI. I would say there probably isn't a direct relation, so SP is one thing and UBI is another. I think that it's possible to develop SP without the necessity for UBI. That's not to say that UBI is bad thing, I think it's a good thing, what I am trying to say is I don't think that SP is dependent upon establishing UBI if that makes sense.

There are lots of SP in other countries where there isn't any UBI in place. Having said that, I think that the course is very interesting to think about whether its possible UBI will help to remedy some of the problems that SP is also trying to tackle. Would UBI help SP be more effective? One may argue that the answer is yes. It's possible to think that SP will benefit from the existence of UBI.

I think that UBI, or its introduction, really does need to be sorted out as part of the wide set of societal changes. We live in a society, whether we like it or not, that has a whole set of values, a value system or value judgement around a whole series of things including a lot around the work and people identities and sense of purpose. I think that the move towards UBI is becoming increasingly important but it's not a panacea that will solve all our problems.

I mean, it is interesting if you think about some of the

community in post-industrialised countries where there is very little work, and to some extent it has been the case for thirty to forty years. So, I am talking about the mining community in Britain. Now, there has been no mining for thirty or forty years, the communities that were still shipbuilding have high levels of unemployment and you could argue that therefore, in these communities, many people have been living on one form or another of social benefit for the last thirty or forty years.

Those are communities who have enforced idleness because there is no work and, in addition, live on benefits which are by no means generous. It pays for your housing; it is very modest money to live on. Now, for a single person it's about £75 a week. It really must pay for everything, except for your housing. Of course, that is not UBI, it's a welfare benefit that you are being given, but its operating like a UBI. It's a guaranteed amount of money. Maybe no longer guaranteed with lots of sorts of sanctions, but what I am trying to say is that communities in Britain where large-scale industry disappeared forty years ago, a high proportion of those communities have not had jobs for the last forty years.

The experience for those communities has not been very good. So, they have welfare benefits, a very modest amount of money to live on and I am quite aware that it's not very much money. You can't live very well with that amount of money. It's probably just enough money to survive on. But, what I am also saying is that you could argue those are communities who have had a lot of time on their hands because there is no work, or very little of it.

However, the results to those communities have not been very good. High levels of ill health, high level of mental ill health and often high level of poor health behaviour, like high levels of drinking, smoking, not eating very good food, partly because of income and not taking exercise very much and also quite a lot of issues around anti-social behaviour, high levels of crime and high levels of drug use. You could argue this causes community breakdown. Now, what I am trying to say is that when we start to think about the shift where we are now to UBI, we also must start making other shifts as well about how we are working with communities, how we are supporting communities, how we are empowering communities, how we are helping communities to think about what's valuable for them and how a community can be more protagonistic in its own destiny and its own decision making.

I guess one of the reasons that people think UBI might be important is because there may be a lot less jobs in the future due to artificial intelligence (AI) and robotics. No one is quite sure yet, but they may have the capacity to destroy thirty percent of the current jobs in Western Europe. Then you think what would they do if their job disappeared even if is twenty percent of workers. Part of the reason for UBI is this idea on how do we de-stigmatise not having a job and do we get people to make more rational decisions about what they want to do with their time and how do we get people to look at time and money very differently to the way we look at it today.

I think that's very exciting and it will require a very different way of valuing what we do. Now, most people who work, the real justification for work is a whole mixture of things, but it's primarily around economic benefits. But, we get a whole lot of other things from work as well. You get companionship from your colleagues, you get a sense of purpose, you get a reason to get up in the morning, wanting to get out of the house, go to work, social contact, all sort of things but we have status in the society, a sense of identity of who we are. All this from going to work, not just for the money.

I think part of the problem is when people have enforced idleness when there isn't enough work for them to do, they lose not just the work and money, but they lose all the other things as well. That's why losing one's job and not being in work is so damaging for people. UBI therefore is only part of the solution around how we ensure that everybody has enough money to live on. But, it's also I think much more important than that, it's about how we start to think about how we use our lives differently and our time differently. I am imagining there might be a lot more people choosing to work part-time maybe to develop other aspects of their life in the remaining time that they have.

I guess you could imagine that if you work in a supermarket filling shelves and you are currently working five or six days a week to earn enough money to live on, if you had UBI, you might say *"Well, I want a little bit more money than my UBI so I might go to work to supermarket for two days week"* because I already get my UBI, but I would like to have a little bit higher level of standard of living so I would work two or three days a week and I will have maybe four days to do things I want to do myself.

How we stimulate people about what they want to do is really important, and how are we able get people to make more choices about what they want to do and how they think about their time differently is really important and exciting. Undoubtedly, coming back to the actual question, what's the relation between UBI and SP. I don't think there has to be a relationship at all and you can certainly do SP without having UBI in place. What I think is at the bottom of your question, which is very exciting, would UBI help people with some of the issue that SP is intending to support. I guess the answer is probably yes, I mean you can think if people had more time in their community and had enough money to be able to live reasonably comfortably, it may encourage people to get involved with a lot more community activities or learning activities, or those where they can express themselves, they could do hobbies and get involved in a whole lot of other things with their community that would be quite meaningful and would support them to feel fulfilled and to feel a sense of learning and pleasure.

However, I don't think it will happen automatically. What I am trying to say is the experiences of some of the regions of Europe, or where there has been very high unemployment for the last thirty or forty years, is that people don't automatically or spontaneously get involved in the activities that are available. An interesting study will tell you that unemployed people are much less likely to use the library than employed people. Now that seems strange if unemployed people have a lot of time on their hand and the libraries are free to use.

You would think that people who are unemployed would utilise libraries more, because they are warm in winter, you are surrounded by other people which is nice, you can borrow books, you can read books, you can sit there and read the newspapers. What happens to people who have become unemployed is that they also become very depressed and they become socially isolated. Then, they stop using even the services which would otherwise benefit them. So, my argument is that yes UBI is going to be very important in the future but we also need to do a lot of other things as well. This is because when people end up with a situation in the next ten or twenty years of considerably increased unemployment – due to AI and robotics – we need to start to think of society very differently, and we need to start to think of society in terms of people, their artistic and cultural expression or sports, leisure activities and all sort of hobbies and past times and this need to become much more central to what we are as a society. Whilst UBI will help, we will need to also think about a lot of other things as well.

With UBI, we also need to think about supporting people to

set up social businesses like social entrepreneurship. I suspect that in the future, we need to think about how we support small economic initiatives around small entrepreneurships. You may need to think about the opportunities for people to make things with their hands like growing food and vegetables, making arts and crafts. Also, within communities, how can we support each other through things like social entrepreneurship and social enterprises, or things like time-banking.

I think those all will be part of this mixture which will also include UBI, and I think that it's going to be very exciting in the future. Hopefully, one that's very empowering and supports people to have a real sense of ownership in their life. If we just think of UBI as giving money to people and they remain to be passive, then that's not going to be very much different to giving unemployment benefits. I see UBI as being part of a whole series of changes like a building block to a brighter future.

It's all going to be about communities and quite small-scale things, which is also interesting because SP often really works at the level of communities as well.

Interview with Steve Howard from Lloydspharmacy

This is his summary on SP

The referral of patients to non-clinical services will become increasingly prevalent, as increasingly we become aware that ill-health is caused by a range of factors . . . socio-economic, poor education, social exclusion, poor lifestyle choices etc., rather than simply organic disease.

The evidence base for the effectiveness of social prescribing interventions is quite limited at present, and the studies I have seen focus on process and inputs rather than outputs, often with no control group. This will need to change to move beyond small sale and niche schemes.

The social value of such schemes needs to be appreciated and quantified . . . reduction in welfare benefits, improvements in social cohesion and mobility as well as the more obvious health benefits should be considered.

The question of who pays is always going to be relevant and particularly so at present in the light of substantial funding cuts in England.

There is no doubt that community referral and social prescribing is aligned to the overall 5YFV, as well as the more recent GPFV, so should be in the thoughts and actions of commissioners.

Effective and evidence based interventions are the key and scalability, and something broader than a small scale local scheme is needed.

Interview with Hala Jawad from Laa Laa

Arun – Hala, have you encountered any patients who have approached you for non-medical reasons? And if so, did you use social prescribing?

Hala – Yeah, quite regularly actually! A lot of people want advice and support with non-medical conditions and feel that their pharmacist is the best person to speak to. For such instances, we use a technique referred to as social prescribing, also known as community referral. This allows GPs, nurses and other primary care professionals to refer people to a range of localised, on-clinical services. There is lots of information provided through both online and offline leaflets and newsletters.

Arun – And what about digital prescribing? Would you consider recommending a mobile app to patients if they were approved by the NHS and MHRA?

Hala – As healthcare professionals, we want to empower the patient to use evidence-based resources and apps which can take pressure of physical care provisions. We don't want to discourage people from contacting a GP or pharmacist if they feel seriously ill, but we do want to use digital technology to educate our patients. There are some fantastic apps out there, such as NHS Choices, Patient.Info & NICE. Some charities also provide some great online learning resources, such as Diabetes UK, the British Heart Foundation and Asthma UK. I'd be happy to point anyone in the direction of evidence-based resources.

Arun – What are your thoughts on patient empowerment strategies, such as giving access to Summary Care Records? (SRCs)

Hala – Personally, I think that all patients have the right to have access their Summary Care Records. As health care professionals, we have a duty to provide a patient centred care to the public, and that should include giving our patients access to their records. This could have positive effects in relation to them taking control of their lives by acknowledging past frailties and help plan for the future.

Arun – In relation to disruptive technologies, what are your thoughts on the Internet of Things (IoT), Blockchains and Artificial Intelligence (AI)?

Hala – I think there's a virtue to the usage of IoT in healthcare as a whole and in pharmacy. IoT encompasses using physical devices which work with each other through an internet connection. For instance, if your Grandmother takes a fall in her house, she can press a buzzer in her home which can alert a carer or ambulance station to her plight. Robot-driven, stock management controls can order medication when they understand that a specific brand or medicine is running low. Automation scares some people, but we should embrace it. Let robots do the legwork while we concentrate on patient care. Artificial Intelligence can help doctors to monitor health developments by entering symptoms onto an advanced piece of software and gain advice and a prescription from a database which gathers information from global sources. As with any online information storage, data protection is of vast importance and we would need to ensure that information is regularly monitored and based on evidence.

Arun – And finally, Hala, do you think that all community pharmacists should become independent prescribers?

Hala – All pharmacists are clinical, regardless of the sector they work in. I can see the future of pharmacist moving toward non-medical prescribing courses. I suppose, the more services that can be provided by pharmacists, the better. Pharmacists are considered as part of healthcare professional team and they are providing more clinical services in GP surgeries or hospitals. So, I can see the future of the community pharmacy quite bright in that regard.

Interview with Karen Harrowing from Quality Systems & Pharmacy Consultancy

Arun – How you would see a national governance framework for SP schemes in community pharmacies, for quality assurance purposes?

Karen – All products and services, whether they are based on pharmaceutical supply or other products and services offered to patients, need to have that governance framework around them. I have previously described the four layers of governance, namely personal level, team level, organisational level and national level e.g. by regulators. Initially, since SP is something which is being worked up more locally (than nationally), those layers of governance will be much more local, and it would be down to the individual professional and professionals in teams working closest with the patient or consumer who are receiving the services to ensure robust governance frameworks are in place.

Like anything else, as it gathers momentum, you would expect to see standards being set by relevant standard bodies.

With SP, I think this will take a bit of time for people to work out what would be appropriate in that space. Ultimately, a regulatory framework may set the principles for SP (not detailed standards). Those principles will mean it will incumbent on individual professionals to follow good practice standards. Traditional organisational frameworks may not be so relevant in the SP and DP arena and so governance frameworks will need to evolve.

Arun – Regarding digital prescribing (DP), as a practical example, the FDA recently set up a Digital Health Unit (DHU) which considers the quality of mobile apps and wearable trackers like the FitBit and Apple Watch. Where do you see it implemented in UK? The NHS has an app store which is in a beta phase, and also the MHRA provides guideline on how to receive the CE marking for mobile health apps. What would be the required steps to make it even more mainstream? For instance, a guideline to follow enabling pharmacists or GPs to prescribe mobile apps to patients.

Karen – I am familiar with the MHRA in terms of the work they are doing into the CE marking of apps to ensure the way that apps are interpreted is effective. So, the CE marking rules would apply for relevant diagnostic apps. Obviously, there is going to be lots of grey areas as the technology develops. I would see that this space may also become occupied with other sorts of accreditation processes over time.

If you look at areas where there have been gaps in standard setting, for example in the cosmetics industry, standards have now been developed. This has ensured that medicines like Botox and the Cosmetic fillers (which are medical devices) are now subject to similar standards for injectable cosmetics.

I know perhaps cosmetic is not the best analogy, but I think there is a similarity in the fact that there have been gaps and new standards have been devised from within the industry, without the need for new regulation.

There may be certain issues that will arise in digital prescribing where people put something into the marketplace which is not potentially effective before more standards are developed that are fit for purpose. People who are keen to demonstrate quality in their products and services will lead the way in this anyway and it will start to create benchmarks.

Arun – There is an increased recognition of VR becoming more mainstream amongst the consumer, there are several start-ups, two in particular from America, one is called MindCotine which is essentially a VR exposure therapy to help the patient reduce their smoking habit, and another one is VRPhysio which shows how to do physiotherapy in an immersive environment at home. There are standards available in America led by the VR/AR Association (VRARA) and Global Virtual Reality Association (GVRA) but I don't think there is one yet in UK. What would be your opinion on making it available in community pharmacy?

Karen – I think, again, sometimes these innovations start to appear before people realise what kind of governance framework is required around them. Some of these areas will start to gather momentum and regulation and standards will have to catch up. Recently the primary care products and services available online have come under scrutiny through CQC inspections, which have demonstrated poor governance and controls. This has created some reaction against on-line services but CQC have also reported on good governance in online services.

I consider some things will attract some negative publicity if they are not set up well. I think that tends to drive calls for improvements – I wouldn't say regulation because I am not sure it is what we need – I think it's about setting standards. If you use the analogy of a physiotherapy app, physiotherapists would not want to have their product effectively tarnished by bad reputation. They would look to put standards around that.

Arun – In your opinion, would it be appropriate for a community pharmacist to teach mindfulness to patients who may be suffering from depression or anxiety? This is to help them improve their wellbeing and if they find it useful, they can follow it up with an experienced mindfulness practitioner or instructor.

Karen – I think the accessibility of community pharmacy is a great advantage for looking at other opportunities in terms of supporting people from a much wider public health perspective. We see mental health issues are increasing rapidly and pharmacies are in a good place to support that. I think the issue that I see is the current way that pharmacies are operating on a supply of medicines basis.

The remuneration and the contractual arrangements have, for a long time, focused on the supply of medicines rather than the benefits in terms of outcomes derived from the skills for other services provided. I think it's also about breaking down the continuing focus on services associated with a supply model in healthy living and public health services, such as smoking cessation. Areas such as Mindfulness, Activity Prescriptions and other SP, directly or VR, are what we need more consultation on. The compensation model based on effectiveness of outcome from actual service delivered with the relevant counselling is going to be more important than supply going forward.

I think community pharmacy is the right location for mindfulness conversations as part of a multidisciplinary team approach to depression or anxiety. The CPPE have been working hard to ensure that pharmacy professionals get consultation skills up to the right levels in pharmacy – we have been trained for a long time with a lot of skills in 'telling'. Pharmacy professionals are good at giving lots of good advice, including on how to take the medicine, but I am not sure that pharmacy professionals are, at this point in time, perfecting their listening skills and hearing what the patient is telling them in a much broader way. Being able to listen to somebody, feedback in order to help them with exercises around mindfulness, is a skill set that many pharmacy professionals still need to develop.

Arun – We can improve the quality of the services delivered by including nutrition, and there is an international qualification in obesity education for HCPs called SCOPE (Specialist Certification of Obesity Professional Education) which is available online. As part of HLP, should it become mandatory for all pharmacies to enable to provide world-class advice around nutrition during MURs?

Karen – I am not familiar with all the community pharmacy contractual arrangements. I am surprised that Health Living Pharmacies are not a contractual requirement at a higher level because I can see there is a huge unmet need at the moment. Community pharmacy seems to be in a very good position to provide healthy living support to people and not only on smoking cessation, alcohol and weight management but, like you say on good nutrition (and exercise), which are so important for healthy lives.

The standards which they would meet would have to seem reasonable for the level of advice they were given. You would potentially have levels of nutritional advice for what you feel competent to give. For example, if you were talking to somebody who had a very straight forward weight loss requirement and who is overweight, then that's one level of advice you could probably give quite satisfactorily with courses such as CPPE.

I think if pharmacy professionals were getting into detailed nutritional information and advice on supplements, they would have more complex training needs. For example, a perpetual weight problem or an eating disorder which had associated mental health issues, that's when your nutritional advice, accompanied with other behavioural information, would probably warrant a more formal education based to the training.

In the UK, professions come under the Professional Standards Authority (PSA), with dieticians being regulated under HCPC and nutritionists having a separate accredited register. For pharmacy professionals they may need to also be on an accredited register if they were looking to call themselves a recognised term to give nutritional advice, e.g. to show they meet the standards for somebody who is using the title of a nutritionist. With Injectable Cosmetics for example, registered Doctors, Nurses and Dentists also demonstrate standards for administration of injectable cosmetic treatments through accredited registers such as 'Treatments You Can Trust'.

It sounds to me that SCOPE is specifically around obesity rather than broad nutritional support. There are other areas that would potentially be helpful in pharmacy because of the increasing obesity to ensure people got relevant nutritional and exercise information.

Arun – Neuroscience practitioners are familiar with neuroplasticity and there is a dedicated academy ran in Australia over nine weeks. Once completed, they receive a certificate if they also pass an online exam and may call themselves a "Brain Science Coach" or "Brain Science Practitioner". I noticed when

I had a few conversations about neuroplasticity with patients during MURs, I was able to highlight the fact that the brain was plastic and that for them to change a behaviour, they need to do it daily, they were much more engaged to take onboard new behaviour because I empowered them with the science behind it.

I have come across pharmacists who aren't familiar with this term. In your opinion, to be able to improve behavioural changes with patients during MURs or face-to-face consultation, should there be a course run by CPPE for pharmacists on the topic of neuroplasticity?

Karen – I think the whole behavioural change arena is daunting for many healthcare professionals who have trained on a treatment and 'medicalised' model of care. My understanding is that neuroplasticity is more about neurons changing, it becomes a physical change which is more around compensating for injury.

In terms of other behavioural science, including NLP, I consider we are going to see it become more core as understanding improves and consumers choose less medicalised options for health and wellbeing. However, we know that patients make choices based on their own risk-benefit assessment, for example the asthmatic who knows that smoking is going to make their asthma worse but is still not motivated to give up smoking when it seems to the pharmacy professional, perfectly logical, that they will have to just stop the activity that makes their health outcome worse. Trying to get to the basis on why they do it and what they get from it, then try to gain their trust to how you can help them requires a deep level of engagement. The whole behavioural / NLP training for healthcare professionals goes hand in hand with the public health agenda.

Arun – Yes, me and my sister, who is a pharmacist too, did the Medical NLP course back in April 2017 and it's different to mainstream NLP and the instructors have been running it since 1996; the founder of Medical NLP is a psychologist and has a clinical advisor who helps him run the course who is a pharmacist and doctor. They teach universities about Medical NLP and they run two courses each year to equip HCPs. I learnt so much content and techniques that I already started to apply what I've learnt in my daily practice for people who are taking anti-depressants.

When I was able to teach them those techniques to help them take ownership of their behaviours, I could see a sudden shift in their body language and the way they behaved. They were extremely grateful at the end of each conversation I had, it only lasted three to four minutes long and that's I am passionate about more people to become involved with Medical NLP. You mentioned the fact that's something not aligned with pharmacy but with public health.

Karen – I think that's a broader piece when people are being prescribed medications. The traditional areas which behavioural support is provided, around smoking, drinking, eating behaviour and so on, fits very well within the public health agenda. That's a more accessible space for pharmacy professionals to start developing Medical NLP skills.

When you start getting into areas around anti-depressant prescribing, you really need to do that within the context of a multi-disciplinary team. For example, if you are in a GP surgery and the prescriber and all those with the duty of care are aware of the conversation.

However, there is potentially a problem applying Medical NLP intervention when medication has already been prescribed for somebody, particularly patients who have potentially complex mental health needs, the pharmacy may not be party to the whole multi-disciplinary team conversation. They should be, and this is where we need to get to, but at the moment, it's not always the case. Community pharmacy professionals are not always part of that team of people who are supporting patients who have many complex needs.

You have obviously done the training around Medical NLP and I consider it would be the start with lifestyle choices that people make. Those are the things that pharmacy can actively get involved in to help create wider conversations with the multidisciplinary team.

I do think SP and DP will gather a momentum, but it's a classic change scenario where you have to have a number of very strong advocates, like yourself, 'change-agents' to get over the hurdles, gain momentum and reduce the barriers of resistance to change. This must get a body of momentum before it starts to become mainstream. I consider that the issue that we discussed around governance and quality standards, need to be established as pharmacy professionals move forward for people to not get caught up in debates on patient safety grounds. This is because, as with any new approach, it only takes one piece of bad publicity for safety concerns to be raised. There may be a tendency to revert to what is known and therefore progress will be slowed.

Embrace the need to establish standards for SP within pharmacy as these standards will improve with time and will create benchmarks and recognition. It will be something that the regulators (e.g. GPhC & CQC) will need to move forward with as well, so professional leadership in good governance and standard setting is vital for SP and DP.

Interview with Gareth Presch from World Health Innovation Summit

Arun – What's your opinion on patient empowerment, by providing them enough information through access of their medical records, so that they can take ownership and make better decisions about their lifestyle?

Gareth – We should be adopting co-design in healthcare (Collaboration). It should be patients and clinicians with shared responsibilities. You should get as much information as possible; we should have access to our records 24/7. We should be able to see everything because this is our information – you have that at the touch of a button.

We can see our bank details in this day and age, but we can't see your our medical records. So yes, I am all up for that. My experiences working with the National Haemophilia Council, was all co-design, working together in collaboration as a team. It works and improves patient safety, it improves the standard of care.

Arun – Yes, this reminds me of SCR which has been rolled out in community pharmacies. At the moment, we can only read the content and we are not able to write new entries. NHS Digital are working towards adding writing access.

Gareth – It's already available to the patient. Dr Amir Hannan in Manchester is giving you full record access through your smart phone. He has been doing it for ten years. We have launched ID SOS which is an electronic card with a unique QR code and you can put your information details on the card in case of an emergency. If you are in a different country or a lone worker and unfortunately, you have an accident, that card can be scanned by the emergency services and they can see whether you are a diabetic or if you have any underlying conditions.

We launched that card and it is currently available on our website idsos.org and it's £12 a year. So those things are happening, the evolution of digital is there and people are taking ownership. It's about community, the majority of healthcare happens in the community. People should have access to their records. Dr Amir Hannan works for NHS England and he is the Chair of WHIS. He has been giving record access for ten years and we need that rolled out nationally and across the world. GPs have the capability to do that, but they need support and help. VR is going to be huge, we are working on multiple projects where VR will help support with education, infrastructure etc. VR is coming.

Arun – What is your opinion on SP?

Gareth – I am aware of SP projects in Manchester and Dublin through St James' hospital. They are currently running SP. It's only a matter of time before it's widely used. It can be used for alternative medicines and therapy as a referral point as well.

In the future, we need to be familiar with dementia awareness and become astute to that, beginning now to promote it. This is because dementia is going to be massive issue and the costs associated with care is going to be huge. We are working on programmes to support early detection.

I am currently working with Julian Gresser in the US on early detection technologies.

Collaborate and we can solve many challenges. If you could do a scan of someone and then be able to see their anatomy through VR – for example: cancer – that level of imagery would be phenomenal.

Community pharmacists could become aware of their role within the community as professionals and how they can alleviate pressure off their GP's acute services which I know pharmacists are already doing. It could be thinking about mental health; how they can collaborate with other agencies and other local community representatives. So the likes of "Mind" (a charity) with a community pharmacy are becoming more of a point of contact and may become akin to GPs in many respects, in terms of their reputation. The GP is the pillar of the community along with your police officer, the pharmacist can be inspired to be at that level. It's building that trust within the community.

Arun – In terms of dementia, again, what are your thoughts on brain exercises? Those developed by companies specialising in neuroscience to help improve the cognitive function of users.

Gareth – I am not an expert in dementia care, but I do read, and I understand that there are benefits in music. Anything that gives you as a patient an improved quality of life equals a positive outcome. I believe in evidence based medicine and make my judgements on science. We are now seeing evidence of other influences that in the past may have been dismissed so we need to have an open mind.

Big Heart Intelligence – It is around the neurological influence of your heart which is a key aspect of stress management and other areas in mental health. These are all emerging technologies, trends, treatments and therapies that community pharmacies should try and incorporate in their day-to-day practice.

Be mindful how you treat each individual that comes into your shop or into the pharmacy, because you don't understand what they are going through or what they have been through today. We all have a game face, your colleagues will have that as well, I am sure they have emotional problems as we are all human. I suppose kindness, understanding and looking it from the other persons perspective, you know and that would help a lot of people.

Arun – Regarding remuneration for SP with the NHS 5YFV, what would be the ideal funding stream? Should it be strictly from the pharmacy budget or can it also come from the social care budget?

Gareth – An integrative model based on collaboration. When you share your resources and intellectual properties, ultimately, you can put as much revenue as you want into something but if you don't have the people then you will not have success.

It's all about the people. Collaboration for me works. I don't have a close enough relationship with the STPs to comment and how the breakdown of the budget is, because I am not in that space. I know from working in the health services that a collaborative approach will end up saving you money. By working together and bring patients into the decision-making and design process is very cost effective.

Arun – Going back to patient empowerment, when you mentioned about people being able to scan QR codes to access information about their health, what are your thoughts on having their health records accessible for data analysis for trends to provide preventative measure for H&W? In 2014, Larry Page did a TED interview and he explained that if everyone shared their medical records, we could save 100,000 lives annually.

Gareth – From my perspective – and I can only speak for my context – I have no problems sharing my information, because it means I will have a better outcome. My experience tells me that if you share your information, you will have a better outcome. Most of our information is out there anyway, when you are on Facebook and Twitter for example.

I was in a supermarket yesterday, when I was going to login in their Wi-Fi and I read the short print, it basically said that they can take all your data and use it if you click "Yes" in the Wi-Fi. So, your data is there and if it's health related, it will have a benefit for you. Especially for chronic illness. I understand privacy and you can put in a mechanism and procedures to ensure confidentiality is in place. Ultimately, if you have a serious accident or if you are involved in any sort of mishap, having your medical record open and present is crucial to make a clinical diagnosis. If you are going to save time and your life, do it.

Arun – Yes, HealthUnlocked offers a similar platform to Facebook but it is aimed at individuals with medical conditions, to meet peers with the same health background. It was shown to have an improvement in their H&W because they were able to discuss it and make better decisions.

Gareth – Peer support is crucial, I worked in haemophilia as the chief officer of the National Haemophilia Council, year on year, we saw improvements because we worked with the patient group and they provided peer support (Irish Haemophilia Society).

Arun – What are your thoughts on nominating a young person to educate the rest of the family on digital technologies, such as mobile apps?

Gareth – That's a good idea and I think you would do it with children to go through the family because they can tell the parents like a knock-on effect. I wouldn't be dismissive of people in their fifties, sixties or seventies as they have a lot to give as they have a lot of experience. I think we should embrace that and we should ask them to be more involved and ask them for more support. They are a generation that we should speak to more and we should learn from because they have a whole life experience and it's very much in the context that we don't tap into that and we should.

Arun – This reminds me of time banking used in the BBBC, where senior citizens can share their experience as they receive support from other people for social inclusion. Do you think there should be a national program for time bank, for those who are socially isolated and especially the elderly, because they can be cut off from society after they reach a certain age? The pharmacist could identify them.

Gareth – This week is volunteer's week. There are 22 million people in the UK who volunteer and this is a resource that the NHS should be tapping into. Why not just ask people to help because they will? You just need to ask, so this is what WHIS is about. It's about having that platform where everyone in society can come together to support the health services. This is exactly what we are about. It's simple, it's not rocket science.

Next week, I have a presentation and it is just one slide, it just shows "community" and all our different activities. All of them are held in health service, every single activity that we do, alleviate pressure off the NHS or globally for the health services. It's just so simple.

Arun – What's our opinion on monthly sessions about different health and wellbeing topics, organised by the pharmacist?

Gareth – To do that, you have to build trust within the community. Historically, we haven't done that very well through our communication. So, you must find out what the community wants, what is their need? Not tell them what they want. It is what do they actually want. Like our approach is today, we are starting a project in Maryport West Cumbria, and I met the local community group six weeks ago, we had a good chat about our work, how we can collaborate and then today, they came and met me, and they have a plan. They want to do something, and I just said yes, we are just supporting them.

Now, they are going to do it with our support which means we build a trust and then we establish a relationship. Then, they stay in control as it's their baby, you see what I mean. It's very powerful because it's them, they control it and it's their community taking ownership. I don't have to tell them anything, we are the cushion because of the WHIS involvement. It will happen overtime because the natural affiliation it becomes with us and then it just grows.

People are more health conscious. Your idea is right, it's spot on but how you approach it, you must think outside of the box. What is that your community is interested in, how do you relate to them and how do you do bridge the gap because you are a pharmacist and they see you as a present authority. You are telling them what to do, that never work. It just doesn't work.

It's not a bad thing but just like you are in school and the teacher tells you to do something and your natural response is to not do it. It's in our nature, like if I tell you, you could do something, you still don't want to do it. Whereas, if I am supporting you and your own ideology comes up with it, you are doing to do it. You see what I mean, it's how you manage and support local peoples and then when you build the trust, then it comes to the point where I am going to look after our H&W. I am not going to have that can of soda, I will just have water and start managing myself a bit better but that will come up over time because there is no silver bullet here. It must take time, it takes trust, everything is trust.

Arun – It remind of patient participatory groups; do you think this should be upscaled?

Gareth – If it works in one place, it can work anywhere. That model is sound, and it consistently delivers safe care.

Interview with
Dr Uli Chettipally from
Kaiser Permanente

Arun – You mentioned the big four as a main focus for aggressive prevention, which lead to a 30% reduction. In your opinion, could those strategies be extrapolated to community pharmacy?

Uli – Yes. To name the four conditions:

1. Smoking
2. Diabetes
3. Hypertension
4. Hypercholesterolemia

These conditions have pharmaceutical products available for treatment. A community pharmacy can be organized to screen, monitor and treat these conditions.

Arun – Being innovation-focused from the start, Dr Umesh Prabhu (from the UK) mentioned that $4 billion were spent in the last 10 years for the IT at Kaiser Permanente (when I had a phone interview with him). Is VR one of the areas of focus for preventative healthcare (e.g. Dr Ralph Lamson's work)?

Uli – We are building the IT infrastructure which includes Electronic Health Records. Once that is fully built and functional, then we can think of additional tools that can be implemented to make the care processes more efficient. VR is currently in its infancy.

Arun – Can Blockchain be used in community pharmacies to help us in the care and wellbeing of the patient?

Uli – Blockchain is a technology that can serve as a backbone for many information systems, where there are trusted users from various entities who need to access the patient information. In that sense, pharmacy can be one of those trusted users.

Arun – IoT as disruptive technology, with the recent NHS hack, by increasing the number of wearable trackers sold in community pharmacy, patients who use it frequently could cause more harm than benefits if it's tampered. Would an AI be beneficial in detecting malicious changes in IoT measurements?

Uli – Systems need to be built that can prevent malicious attacks, whether it is AI or otherwise. Devices being connected to the system need to have the same protections and safeguards as sensitive patient data.

Arun – Do you have any other thoughts where disruptive technologies can benefit patient health and wellbeing in community pharmacies?

Uli – A community pharmacy can play an important role in managing chronic conditions. In the future, AI systems will be able to recommend treatments based on patient characteristics, and the community pharmacy will be able to monitor the response to such treatments. A community pharmacy can also play a role in screening for risk factors and immunizations.

Interview with Prof Joseph Proietto from SCOPE

Joe – SCOPE is based around obesity rather than nutrition. They are slightly different things.

Arun – Most patients have an LTC and many of them have a large BMI, including obesity. It includes co-morbidities like diabetes and some are smokers. I personally feel that the SCOPE course will greatly enhance our skills in helping patients. There are 1.8 million daily visits to community pharmacies with around 44,000 pharmacists in this sector. Should all community pharmacists do the course, with the option to refer patients to a dietician if needs be.

Joe – Here in Australia a lot of people seek advice from community pharmacists. I am sure, it's the same in UK, so it would be useful for all pharmacists to give advice that is evidence based and up-to-date about obesity. I think it would be a good idea for the pharmacists to up-skill themselves about recent work around obesity. The SCOPE course is going to change significantly in October 2017, in that there will be a core pathway which will result in the student being more confident in managing obesity.

Those who have done the Scope course before may see one or two of the previous modules that have been included in the core pathway, but most of it will be newly written. We will have links from the core pathway to the other modules as background information. All of that should be able to give the person who does the course, a good grounding on obesity to give more evidence-based advice.

Arun – I personally feel having a dedicated pathway to refer a patient to a dietician would be hugely beneficial. Especially with the fact that obesity is leading problem worldwide. Should obesity campaigns in collaboration with public health be promoted in community pharmacies?

Joe – Given the exposure that the population has to a pharmacy, it's a good source of information about the condition. For example, as you see from the module on the causes of obesity, what appears to be self-evident that obesity is caused by lifestyle problems is not true. Obesity is predominantly genetic. I think pharmacists are well positioned but the referral path shouldn't stop at the dietician because it will be eventually necessary that the patient goes and see their GP as medication may be needed to maintain weight loss.

This is because as you see from the module on body weight regulation, most people who lose weight, regain weight and now we know why. That needs to be propagated to everybody and pharmacotherapy is necessary for weight maintenance. It's not just weight loss.

Arun – Are there any plans to include malnutrition as part of the current module? Or will it be in a different course? This becomes relevant in care homes and anorexic women.

Joe – Nutrition is an important issue when you are asking people to either lose or gain weight. We don't have any module on anorexia because we deal mainly with obesity. I run an obesity clinic, we use very low energy diet to improve nutrition in people who are losing weight.

We've shown that you should use VLCD (very low-calorie diet) like Optifast or Optislim, you can lose weight without being malnourished. It does not require a dietician's specialised knowledge. The dietician is trained to provide a balanced diet which means that the diet of the dietician gives you will ensure that you have all your micro-nutrients. That's the skill of the dietician. If you are doing the weight loss phase with VLCD, you don't need the dietician because they get all their vitamins in the very low energy diet (VLED).

When you need a dietician is when you are coming off the diet and going on to ordinary food. This is how we use a dietician in my clinic. When you are going to ordinary food, it would be useful to know how you should structure your meals so that you get all your micronutrients once you stop taking the supplements.

Arun – From what I've learned at BBBC, it's easier to revert from obesity as a child than as an adult. In your opinion, should we go more upstream by educating local schools on the topic of obesity?

Joe – You will need to speak with the parents on the topic of obesity. Talking to the teachers and headmasters is not a problem but they are already aware of this problem, so I don't think it would be a good avenue for your efforts. Speaking to the children themselves, is not a good thing to do because you end up potentially increasing bullying and things like that.

Arun – Should we use VR as a medium of education with patients to help them retain information for longer?

Joe – I have no knowledge in using VR as a form of education. I spend a lot of time educating my patients and I also wonder how much do they retain but because of that, I have written a book. You may want to look that up, it's called "Body Weight Regulation – Essential knowledge to lose weight and keep it off" published by Xlibris, you can order it online (it is available on Kindle).

We need to mobilise everybody who has contact with the population to educate them about the true nature of obesity as you will read in the book. I think that community pharmacies are very well positioned to do that as well as GPs.

Interview with Garner Thomson and Dr Khalid Khan from The Society of Medical NLP

The Society of Medical NLP was founded in 1998 by Garner Thomson with the support of Dr Richard Bandler, co-creator and developer of Neuro-Linguistic Programming, and Dr Khalid Khan as clinical advisor.

Official website: www.medicalnlp.com
Facebook: The Society of Medical NLP

The Pharmacist can exacerbate the patient medical conditions through priming and anchoring when doing Medicine Use Reviews (MURs) and New Medicine Service (NMS) as we also follow a tick box online form, similarly to GPs. This can be overcome by doing the Medical NLP course, but most pharmacists are unaware of NLP in general.

Arun – For those who do buy your amazing book, and are waiting to do the 7-day course, what preparation do you recommend them to do until then?

Garner – The "Magic In Practice" book is a very good primer and my suggestion is people open their mind on what's happening when they read the book. If they feel confident, they can try some of the techniques, nothing wrong with that, but in reality, they won't become the solution if they don't have the guidance to do it.

Khalid – Remember we talked about beginner's mind at the beginning (this was at the start of a recent Medical NLP 7-day course), so, yes, keep the mind open.

Community Pharmacy shop floors are filled with planograms of medical conditions which can worsen the symptoms of patients by priming the unconscious mind (the Nocebo Effect). There are currently no health and wellbeing planograms except from vitamins and weight loss ones.

Arun – What should be the recommended ratio of planograms between medical conditions and health and wellbeing in the shop floor? When I developed the MP Model with Ying and Yang back in November 2016, I thought of a 50:50 ratio.

Garner – I feel that it can be 100 percent, the point is we want to be selling health to people, rather than disease, or, disease-management, in any form. It's a challenge. A little while ago, when I was working in a practice in Scotland to teach a course there, they were very proud of their new department in hospital – the "pain" department. I was introduced to everybody called "pain" doctors, "pain" psychologists, "pain" nurses and so on. Everything emphasised suffering. The challenge is to reframe it in ways that are more positive. If you can't think of anything else to look at it, call it "pain relief" until you can find a better definition.

Arun – The main source of income for community pharmacies is from dispensing prescriptions and the other source from sales made in the shop as an additional source of income. This remind me of the work done by Kari Modén from Stockholm Design Lab for Vardapoteket (the Swedish pharmacy chain). She designed the pharmacy to have artworks almost as form of education for patient visiting the premises, so it didn't feel like a pharmacy at all. Also, the number of sales in that pharmacy increased by 30 percent and won 4 additional services from the local council (like CCGs). There is definitely a scope for 100 percent health & wellbeing planograms.

Garner – The use of positive ideograms acts a primer. However, the kind of pictures and posters used in pharmacies now are quite grim.

Arun – Another example I can think of is Bromley-By-Bow Center (BBBC) where I went to an open-day in February 2017, and the surgery doesn't look like one at all. The walls are wooden with great pictures. I also went to the Social Prescribing Conference in May 2017 where one of the speakers was from BBBC (Sir Sam Everington OBE) and confirmed the health recovery was higher than Kaiser Permanente in USA.

Garner – Always remember that there are people whose vested interest is in creating a negative response. The concept of creating anxiety in someone and then selling their products to reduce their anxiety is a well-known but cheap marketing technique. We must think in terms of providing health, all of us. The work you are doing is very valuable. You also talked about annual stress vaccinations . . . a very good idea which needs to be recognised by other pharmacists like you.

Most patients have a smartphone and get into a "trance" when using it as, they become engaged to it through habit.

Arun – It was only possible thanks to your book which greatly opened my mind. I strongly believe every pharmacist should be a Medical NLP practitioner. What are your thoughts on mobile health apps to implement more useful habits? (e.g. healthier diets, better quality of sleep, meditation, etc . . .)

Kalid – It's a good idea. as people are much healthier having the power of the mobile phones. We are getting useful results already. Of course, it depends on the app and the outcomes they measure.

Garner – The point many developers do not really understand what has to be done and just push their products on the market, using buzz-words like heart rate variability (HRV). Many apps do not measure HRV at all; what they show is heart rate, resting pulse rate et cetera, but they are simply rebranded as something they are not. So, I think there are two classes of app, one of them is connects your vitals with the doctor, and these can be very useful. Many apps measure downregulation of people's health and condition, and I think we should reverse that. What we should have is more apps encouraging people to do better, apps that to measure the level of their health and well-being. This is what we are currently working on at the moment.

Arun – I read 2 books from Dr Bertalan Meskó (The Medical Futurist) where he did several reviews of health apps and devices. One of them is called *The Muse* which is a headband which measures your brain waves to help recognise if you are in a stressed or calm state.

Garner – This is true and there are several of them. The thing we must **remember** is that the quality varies dramatically. Very often what these things are measuring is not brain waves but skin conductivity. Generally, skin conductivity is a fairly basic measurement of stress. To get a very good reading, we need quite complex equipment, not just a headband. I am still looking for easily available equipment that is going to give a proper reading. The other thing is this. My feeling is people don't need to be told when they are stressed but how to get out of it—or, even better, how to cope with or avoid it. There is something called neurofeedback which measures the level of the autonomous system. That's where HRV come in. We use that in treating some of our patients, especially children. We have a very nice software for kids such as a digital colouring book to teach them to manage their states. Another one is connected to a balloon to rise for a trip to cross the countryside which is achieved by modifying their states. It's all getting very exciting.

Arun – Many companies are bringing chatbots to answer medical queries, do you think having these on their phone will remove the human touch?

Garner – Yes, always. What we are very much about is about self-efficacy; chatbots can be useful up to a point. But, there is an issue where the control is outside of the person and diminishes self-efficacy. The other things we noticed with apps is that people start very well with them and then stop using them. Whereas what we want to do is to install a good response and a good state.

Arun – This would be to install the gamification spirit, like a reward system, in the game. For example, Walgreens offer a "Balance Rewards" program where patients receive points for healthy choices such walking, weight tracking and measuring blood pressure. Those points can be then redeemed at the pharmacy.

Garner – But you know, if you read books by Dan Ariely, you will find that people are generally not motivated by money or points or things like that. It sounds that they should be, but they are not. So, we need to find other ways of motivating. New behaviours and new practices like breathing require practice, and people need to be encouraged to do this. There already are very useful apps like one called "MotivAider" which we started using way before apps were available on other devices. This can be set at any time and duration, you wish, and it will buzz to remind you of your posture or to breath properly or to do whichever things you set it for. It's a very simple thing to use and is very useful.

Arun – So this is like a primer to anchor an action?

Garner – Absolutely, we are doing it already. For example, how many people feel buzz in their pocket and they think it's their phone but its' not their phone at all? This is a known phenomenon where people are learning a new neurological response. We want people to learn responses that support healing and health.

Arun – The NHS have a developed an app store for approved apps which meets the required standards and the MHRA also developed the CE marking for tested apps. This is almost like a stamp of quality. Do you believe The Society of Medical NLP should have a similar certification process for mobile app meeting the required standards?

Garner – We very much would like to do that. What we would like is to measure is how well something works inasmuch as it hands over efficacy to the user. The only apps I approve of are ones that you no longer need after a short while. They will train you to get rid of them.

Social Connectedness is important to improve health.

Arun – Do you think social prescribing should become mainstream to complete the "ritual"?

Khan – That's a brilliant idea, we are doing it already and the community pharmacy is an ideal place to do this. We are in a very good position to enable social connectedness.

Garner – The NHS has tried that without much success. At one point they gave people gym memberships, but it just didn't work because I think there was not enough patient-friendly information, whereas pharmacists have a much more personal relationship and consultations that last longer than 5 to 8 minutes. You are in a great position to do this.

Travel and Flu vaccinations are done by community pharmacists. WHO recognises "stress" as an epidemic but there are no therapies currently offered in community pharmacies.

Arun – What are your thoughts on Annual Stress Vaccinations (ASV) using Medical NLP techniques?

Garner – I love this idea because I don't agree with the current view of treating people for "stress" as if it is a thing that exists outside the person. We find out what's causing you stress, stop it and try to get it to go away. In reality, people who have all the stressors removed get worse, and that's why when they are given time off from work they very often deteriorate. That's because what's missing is not stress but the ability to cope with the challenge. So, we want people to develop resilience.

Arun – Is there anything you would like to add?

Garner – Yes, one of the GPs on your course (I did it in April 2017) said to me that she has a patient that had been referred to her as she had an uncontrollable itching. Everything that she tried didn't work so what they decided is that it was all in the mind as though it was separate from the body. The GP asked her where she felt comfortable and worked to expand that comfort rather than trying to fight it. She had a positively good result on that. So, it's always important to move ahead towards healing and health as opposed to trying to remove disease. We see a pro-active approach that was salutogenic, that's the big thing, if there was a single message in all our work that is it.

Arun – In terms of VR, the reason I included it as part of my book is there is an app called Sno-World in USA. It is used in burns victims where the pain threshold was reduced by up to 60% in comparison to morphine with no risk of addiction. With VR Therapy applications in pharmacies for people who are finding it very hard to visualize like for the Swish Pattern, would having a VR app to facilitate this process be useful?

Garner – That's one approach and that app you are talking about is using hypnosis since that's the underlying principle of how it works. The problem with that is that the research they have done is limited but yes at the same time, they got the results out of it. Since there is no control by the person delivering the imagery, it's just an app. It's the same thing that happens when you are in a hypnotic state. Some people get results from that and other people not. But if you are sitting in front of someone, I can start to talk to you, I can change the tone of my voice, use nodding, asking questions to see how relaxed you can become. So, I can feedback using you with varying states – that's the difference; I think it's good but limited.

Arun – How about using VR as a method of education, rather than therapy?

Garner – I think VR and AI generally are already being used. I am curious to see what happens because we know that the structure of people's brains change whenever they are exposed to the internet. If they are exposed for any length of time to VR, I am curious to see what happens. I expect it to be a double edged-sword. I think it can be very useful but on the other sense, it could be instant psychosis where people have difficulties in distinguishing what's real and not.

Interview with Grainne from Heartfulness

Grainne – The way I came to meditation was motivated by wanting to live a better life and wanting to be proud of who I have become. The feeling that life is not just about what you earn, what you have in your hands, what you can pass on to your children, it's really about who you become.

Meditation invites a silent language with what is deeply pure within each person. It is a search for that warmth and love within yourself and then realising it is possible to learn this new quiet language and interpret its messages to enable you to live a fully active, involved, joyful and happy life. It becomes a living inner warmth which over time builds resilience and as that increases, so does your capacity for openness to all that you encounter daily. People come to meditation for all kinds of reasons, usually they have had difficulty or disillusionment in their lives and they are searching for something deeper.

Many of us live our lives in search of love and acceptance, be that by holding tightly to others, or gathering wealth or status. The next thing you must do is protect what you have gained or achieved and even to increase it in order to maintain a sense of safety, acceptance and therefore love. What if you allowed yourself some time to discover that place in yourself, which is love itself?

Here is what might happen, you can still do everything you are doing but you are no longer so fixated on the outcome. You are then free to participate in your life with joy, openness and relaxation and conversely this makes the achievement of tasks a much easier process. The connection you make during your morning meditation changes your inner state and has a positive effect on everything you interact with during the day. Have you ever come home from work and noticed one of your family members is in a bad mood? Gradually, over the course of the evening, others can become effected by it. We have all experienced these things; we are affected by one another in more ways than we care to believe. When you meditate over time, you begin to find the very best in yourself and that's what you bring into your day, that's what you share with others and that profoundly changes your experience of life.

A representation of everyday life could be like the sea. On top, there are sailing boats, speedboats, everything going on – wind, rain, clouds and sunshine. Really, meditation is like taking a breath and dropping down beneath that water so that you find yourself in a place that is much quieter. You are still in the sea (and a part of life) it allows time and space to recharge so that you can return to the surface relaxed and refreshed.

When you come back up to the surface that quietness lives on in you and you can be on top of the sea with the rain, the hail, the sunshine, all those things; but somehow inside yourself there is a continuing connection to the quietness warmth and love. From there, you can live your life and make your decisions and that inner quietness that is increasingly present begins to affect the people and things around you.

This quietness, warmth, love is not something esoteric, strange amazing, it is simply our inner state and it applies to everyone. The only real difference between one person and the next is how deeply it has become buried. So, when you start it can be like digging a well, firstly its rocks and boulders they you reach damp soil, then the sludgy mud and finally the water comes, crystal clear water! Meditation is like everything in life; all the worthwhile things require some effort.

It is rather counter-intuitive in our modern-day life to "do nothing", it's like: what will I gain from doing that!? When Buddha was meditating for all those years, people said to him, *"So what did you gain from meditation?"* he said, *"Nothing, but ask me what I have lost? I have lost fear, anger and hatred"*.

The first misconception about meditation is you are "doing" nothing you are in fact watching and developing a sensitivity, learning a language so gentle and subtle that is opens you up to another whole aspect of yourself. I was a person who disliked myself, and despite having an amount of worldly success I could not find connection or peace. I used my skills and abilities to chase dreams, moved around the world, worked for others, build businesses, but in the end, none of these things were as fulfilling to me as I had hoped. I kept asking myself, "is this what it is all about?" Is life nothing other than gathering stuff which I ultimately must leave behind? So, despite so called success, I continuously felt something was missing.

I decided to go searching and looked at many practices over many years and even travelled to India. As soon as I found Heartfulness, which was in my town, and sat for mediation. I knew I had found what I had been searching for, one of the reasons I like Heartfulness is because it is empowering. Having come from an Irish Catholic background, I was drawn to its openness and spirit of enquiry, it helps you to gain mastery over yourself. No one is going to tell you what to do, what you should do, what you should become; but you begin to develop a conversation with yourself about those things. So, you return to your authentic individual self and decide what that is going to be. You become your own Master and Master of your destiny. That takes a certain amount of courage, because it means taking personal responsibility for yourself and your life. I did see a quote once outside a restaurant that read "Be yourself, everyone else is taken". This journey of meditation is the grandest adventure without ever leaving home and it is also about returning to your authentic self.

Of course, it doesn't have to be the grandest biggest thing, it is just that for me it was. What I love about the Heartfulness practice is you can approach it from many different levels. Some people do it, simply to relax – they are feeling stressed in their lives and they want something to provide relief; it works for that. Others do it because they want to focus better, and improve their performance at work; it will work for that too. Other people do it because they want more personal development at many levels including the spiritual; and it works beautifully for that also. I would say take none of this to be true and if you are interested I invite you to have a go and make your own judgement.

There are a few things we do in Heartfulness that makes us different from other forms of meditation, and they also make it a very effective practice. Even people who have been meditating for years come to experience it and are perhaps still searching for something deeper. Our Heartfulness practice uses something called *pranahuti* which is an ancient yogic energy, for the transformation of man. It is difficult to explain and much more easily to experience. It is completely free to learn and available to everyone. Every trainer that helps others does it for free; there will never be a charge for it because how can you charge for something that is priceless? So, no one gain's anything by you meditating. I like this approach because it feels somehow clean. "I have tried this, it works very well for me, come and try it". I pass it on because it is wonderful, I do not sell it.

You can take it at any level you want and build up gradually in a way that suits you. This practice that has been simplified to suit modern man, there is no special pose, no special mantras; you simply sit in the comfort of your home, so that you can forget about your body and imagine light in your heart. Initially, it takes a few sessions with a trainer to become familiarised with the practice.

Once you do those three to four sessions, of half an hour each, you can meditate more deeply on your own. The reason why it's called Heartfulness is because the heart encompasses the essence of a person. We often say, 'a warm-hearted person' or a 'cold-hearted person'. We work on the heart as it is central to a person's being and the Heart being central, gradually effects all other areas of the body, it brings calmness and gradually quietens the mind. Heartfulness is not attached to any religious organisations or denomination and is recognised by the United Nations (UN) in more than hundred twenty countries around the world.

The second part of the practice and just as important as the meditation, is the cleaning process. During our lives, we take in impressions through our senses; we are bombarded with information, images, and thoughts every day, all day. Those things are like energy waves passing through our bodies and they can cause patterns within us and make us act in a certain way. We then take actions based on these busy thoughts, leading at times to less than satisfactory outcomes. In our practice, they are called *samskaras*, patterns that build up over time leading us to act in a particular way, almost without choice.

To counteract this, we do cleaning at the end of every day. This means sitting in the evening when you return from work or your day is over and imagine light coming into our heart and all the impressions of the day flowing out the back. It means that you physically offload our day. You don't have to think about what transpired, good or bad but just imagine it leaving your body along your spine. It is like when you get into the shower you simply wash, you do not examine each speck of dirt to remember where it came from; you wash and come out clean and refreshed. The evening cleaning has the same effect on your mind and body; you will feel refreshed.

Now with the cleaning, we have an opportunity to return to any problems the following day with an entirely fresh approach. It avoids you becoming so deeply absorbed in difficulties that you become enmeshed in them. This can easily happen – to give a simple example, in to-days world where we are subjected to images of the perfect physical form, how to look, what to wear, an acceptable shape, self-acceptance is something we struggle with more and more. One of the things that really drew me to this practice was that, right from the start, the first step is about just that, self-acceptance. It is a very vital part of our personal transformation; without it we are stuck in judgement of ourselves and invariably others. It becomes more difficult to develop love for ourselves, never-mind for somebody else. Without these basic things, it is easy to become disconnected with the people around you and disconnected with your world. You can fall into this dark space which is what lots of people experience. Self-acceptance is the very first step that meditation can give you: the ability to be compassionate towards yourself, to gently understand yourself and then find the courage to change in a way that is more helpful to who you wish to be.

So, we have talked about how the practice can help physically, by stress reduction and aiding sleep, mentally by helping you to focus, solve problems and change. If you look at it from a spiritual perspective, we can glimpse its ultimate value. It is well documents that we as human beings, have a baseline consciousness which we use to navigate our daily lives, work, family & recreation. Below this lies our sub-conscious, which again is well documented by the various sciences, this holds an enormous amount of information including everything that has ever happened to us. Above our base line conscious lies our super-consciousness state, where intuition, inspiration and wisdom exist. Meditation when done correctly begins to expand your baseline consciousness up into the super-consciousness and below into the sub-conscious.

That means within your expanding conscious realm, you start to have more sensitivity and intuition which enables you to fully live your life and make more cohesive decisions. It also helps you to experience others in a deeper and more compassionate way. Without doing anything more, than sitting for half an hour morning and evening you begin to develop a loving acceptance of yourself and others and to experience life in a more meaningful way.

Our minds, like our devices, have become busier and busier over time; massive amounts of information flow through them and as a result, they have nearly gone into overdrive. If you ask anyone to feel their mind, they can do it in an instant but if you ask them to feel their heart, it is generally not as easy. Since the heart is the centre of the body and it pumps blood to everywhere within the body, it affects all the organs. So, without engaging the mind, the heart will and can calm it down. In Heartfulness, we don't concentrate on the mind; we concentrate on the heart, which has a much greater magnetic field than the mind. You can with your heart affect other people much more easily than with your mind.

Meditation does require a degree of self-discipline. Like anything in life, you don't become a fantastic guitar player or gymnast without practice. To meditate is to think of something continuously, we have all mediated about things in our life, we often, for example, meditate on our problems. You don't just jump on a bike and start pedalling around, initially it takes some effort. It's not difficult to learn to meditate and once you do, you will never forget but it does take a little bit of time initially. I would say it is time extremely well spent.

I think what I have experienced with people and myself in my practice it that you become more tolerant of so many things. We just don't get angry anymore. It profoundly affects our ability to be happy in the world, to be joyful. Not in a way that is artificial, but just in a quiet way – for so many beautiful things – and it is easy to appreciate them when you are not in a spiral of *"me, myself and I"* or in a spiral of your own perceived problems.

It's not that the problems aren't there, it is that you are not as connected with them or triggered by them as much as you would otherwise be. You also have lots of skills and tools at our disposal to help work through them. Surrender is simply noticing what is happening without having a hissy fit about it. When your triggers are being reduced all the time your resilience increases, and your ability to cope with difficulties also increases. When we have this expanded approach, difficulties dissolve much more easily, then they would in the past. I think a hugely beneficial aspect of meditation: is simply the ability to be content and to live a good life.

Meditation doesn't stop us having a full family life, working for a living and having a busy and active life. This is what I love about the practice – it's not for monks, not for people who must go away for weeks at a time. It's half an hour in the morning when everyone is asleep, half an hour in the evening and a thought before sleep. It is accessible to everybody, no matter what you do. It is usually for people between the ages of 16 to 116!

Arun – Is there any reason for this minimum age requirement?

Grainne – A younger child may do Heartfulness so they can learn to be in touch with their heart. Meditation is a powerful practice and you must have a fully formed body and mind for it. It is also good for people to come to it of their own volition and not because their mother or father pushes them towards doing it. So, you need to be a certain age and level of maturity before undertaking this practice.

Arun – Would it be best for the person to do the face-to-face training first before using the app?

Grainne – Yes, I think so, there is an app and a website. We are in 120 countries around the world and there are trainers in all those countries, almost in every city. You can go on to the website, and it will put you in touch with a trainer, all for free. Where ever you are in the world you can meditate with a trainer via the app. There are groups, in most cities around the world, you can go and meet with that group and learn to meditate with them. If you are far away from a local group, you can still do your own practice at home and a have a trainer available online or over the phone to help you. There are many ways to access Heartfulness. It is on tap all the time, in any way, shape or form that is most convenient to you.

Arun – I did the session with you and I found it extremely valuable. In your opinion, should pharmacists be able to refer patients to Heartfulness sessions?

Grainne – Yes definitely, disease which shows in the physical body often has its source in the feelings and emotions. The health benefits of Meditation are now well documented. Anybody who is over the age of sixteen can start and improve their mental health and wellbeing.

Arun – You mentioned that you went to India. Was it to receive more knowledge about Heartfulness?

Grainne – I always believed that the divine existed. Being brought up as a child in Ireland with Catholicism, they presented a view of God, and, in a way, I just could not believe. Even as a child, I could not believe it because I would look around the world and I would see kittens, puppies & children and so many amazing beautiful things. I couldn't believe that the God they told me about who was supposed to be tough and unforgiving, could be that and yet make such beautiful things. So, I chose to have my own idea of God based upon my experience.

When I was older I went in searching, I remember making the prayer, that if you are e real, let me find you. Growing up in Ireland I knew nothing of any other religions, we were certainly not told about them in school and this was the days before the internet. I looked at lots of different things Buddhism, Sufism the Hindu religion and Gurus in India. Nothing was right; nothing answered my question I couldn't say what it was I was looking for, I just knew I would know when I found it. The minute I sat down for Heartfulness meditation I knew my prayer had been answered.

I have been doing it daily for fifteen years and there is still so much more to learn. Neuroscience is now able to measure the effects of meditation on brain patterns and prove its benefits. There are many people out there that don't believe something unless science can validate it. Meditation is something people have done for thousands of years; it is wonderful that finally science is able to prove its value. So those who needed proof, also have a way in. It is possibly the most productive thing you can do in your life.

Arun – Do you have any advice for pharmacists to embrace Heartfulness, or any other related activities based around meditation? Including having a trainer to run sessions inside the pharmacy or surgery to reduce the distance gap?

Grainne – I would be very happy to come to a pharmacy conference and talk to pharmacists about meditation and let them experience it for half an hour. Knowing it can only come from experiencing it – not hearing regurgitated facts – pharmacists are in a position to be able to help signpost people to more holistic approaches as well as dispensing medication. The Heartfulness solution is free, all-encompassing and the only side effect is well being. Sometimes issues or illness comes into our life to wake us up and invite us towards another more holistic path. Pharmacists do have the opportunity to signpost people towards authentic ways to live a richer happier life and I would encourage them with all my heart to fully utilise this potential.

Interview with Devin C. Hughes from Diversity Advantage LLC

Arun – Many people get mindfulness and meditation confused. I would like to know your opinion, as an expert, in this area to help define what the main differences are between mindfulness and meditation.

Devin – Meditation is a practice which you can exercise with. In contrast, mindfulness, in this context, work along differently. You think what you can do to reset the brain or depress it and pulse positive emotions. For some people, mindfulness might be, for example pharmacies where you will be busy checking meditations all day, it can be very hectic, very stressful and play kind of catch up, so mindfulness might be taking two, three, five to ten seconds to reset your emotions, just to remind the brain again good things are happening. It's the attention of being mindful which just doesn't happen. Most of us are either worried about what happen or what's going to happen, then never taking time of enjoying what is happening.

Arun – So being in the present, in terms of scalability, what would be time-frame needed to teach somebody who hasn't done mindfulness before, to build their confidence to then be able teach it to other patients, or refer them to a mindfulness practitioner? What is your opinion?

Devin – So there are two parts. Part of it is wherever I am in the world and you can maybe concur, most of us as human beings are not taught those skills. This is something we must learn so to answer your question specifically, it's an inside out proposition. It starts with me and then I can share it with others. Typically, what I find to teach mindfulness practice, it must become a habit. So, I must do something intentionally everyday just like when I brush my hair, put deodorant and brush my teeth because the brain like structure as part of neuroscience. The thing the brain seems to do every day intentionally, it starts to automate those processes. So, I help people or assisting whomever, create the structure of making mindfulness practice a habit.

Arun – So it will depend on how quickly they are able to formalise neurologic pathways in their brains before it becomes a habit. So, they can start to feel confident to then share it with patients or other people.

Devin – Yes, I take a step further. Let's say me and you are working on mindfulness practice. What I will do is pair you and I up, so I get people a partner, so I can support you and you can help support me which gets further to develop a habit. We know certain things are good for us, but we don't do it. We should eat right, we should exercise but we don't do it. The reason why is because we are getting lots of stuff. When I pair you up to you or an individual plan and then I create an opportunity for you to help each other develop that, to become a habit.

Arun – In your opinion, is it best to do this training face-to-face, or can it be completed online? Which do you think is the most efficient way of helping somebody to reach that habit of mindfulness.

Devin – I have a bias towards face-to-face, if I can see you, or whatever that is, but with Skype, there are things that I can check in with you to see how you are doing. It's not to you, it's for you. So, either one, face-to-face is better but this works too.

Arun – Before you teach somebody mindfulness like, in our case before we can refer them to a mindfulness practitioner, should there be a set of criteria that patients must tick first before referral or suggest to do mindfulness to help them?

Devin – There are a couple of things, number one, anytime you ask someone to change and you introduce them to a new behaviour, you need to explain to them at least why. Why me, why this, why now, why does it make sense, give them a context. This is because what I found is if you come to me and ask me to start doing this and I never heard of this from anyone, I get suspicious. Why are you telling me to do it, are you saying that I am unhappy, I have bad attitudes, I start getting that. So, you need to tell people the why it's good for you, good for your wellbeing, good for your health and those are all sort of things you can do that don't take that much time, it will make you feel better, you can share it with friends and family.

Then, proactively show them this, it doesn't take that much time and show how every little thing they can do throughout their day consistently, what will create big benefits health-wise and wellbeing-wise.

Arun – In terms of the aspects of running mindfulness, what is the best proposed activity? Do they just use communication, or do they have to do tasks at home like writing a diary on things you should be reminded on what's happening right now to forcefully focus their mind on the present?

Devin – In the beginning, the brain needs, what I call triggers, reminders and alerts. Most people have one of these. I have people putting it on their calendar, some people have sticky notes. If you think about it, over the next 21 or 24 days, what can you do overall to remind yourself to get up to do this every single day. You can literally put it in your calendar, have an alert at 8am every morning before I go to work or at 12 o'clock, instead of eating my lunch by myself in the pharmacy, I will go for a walk so to get some exercise.

It will be very intentional to provide some structure and alert. You can even have your partner to agree with you, you may say *"Hey, I am best in the afternoon. So, Devin, I want to check in with me at 4pm every day to see if I have done it. If I haven't, then could you check in again."* It's all about the accountability rule in the process.

Arun – So, you are empowering the person to take ownership of the mindfulness practice.

Devin – Yes, by virtue of helping them, it also helps you because if I see you succeeding, then my brain begins to recognise that I am going to continue to do it too.

Arun – Like a feedback mechanism where if you succeed, you are doing the right techniques and the right words are being used for them to enable that change. In terms of environment, can anybody do it anywhere no matter how noisy it may be, or does it need to be in a quiet environment which is very tidy?

Devin – I think certainly it's a little bit easier if it's not as hectic or busy but quite often I do it in the airplane, at the airport, I do it when I travel, when I close my eyes, it kind of reset my brain on what's going on around me. Especially if I am feeling a little bit stressed. So, I think sometimes, in environment where it's really hectic, it's almost more needed. It just kind of reset the brain because too often, we try to multitask and that's not possible. It's an easy thing you can do regardless of where you are.

Arun – In terms of all the possibilities of mindfulness, are there any contraindications for its use, like criteria for people to avoid it because of personal mental health problems. For instance, those who suffer from psychosis, would mindfulness be a problem for teaching them, are there any risks for certain patients? Or is it open to everybody?

Devin – No, it's open to everyone and mindfulness has been around for thousands of years. We just have not had the science to substantiate it to clearly show that its good for us so it's open to everyone. How you do it certainly is up to you for example when you tend to meditate. Being in the very present, not attached the network within. If I am in New York city and I work, I will have 8 hours to meditate a day because I have a job. Its situational also depending on where you are, if you are a single mother, or a mother with children, it's going to be hectic regardless of where you are in the situation.

Arun – For lifestyle habits, would somebody's quality of sleep and diet affect the quality of the mindfulness habit?

Devin – Certainly, it would be easier for you but in some cases, I know people who were sleep deprived. They just can't get a good night sleep, they are restless and that's actually helped them to self-rewind their mind down. Too often, people think mindfulness is about controlling one of your thoughts which is not possible. We don't control our thoughts, but we can be mindful being very consciously of the thoughts we are having. Why do I keep having this recurring thought or whatever that is? It's an interesting knowledge in that and we are kind of resetting our brain with what those things are.

Arun – For language barriers, let's say to communicate effectively, the second person must speak the same language. How would you approach somebody who doesn't speak English, for example? Would you ask for an interpreter to communicate in between or would you emphasise more on body language and movement of your hands to portray the intended actions to take?

The context of that question is that some people who come into a pharmacy may be from a different country like Poland or China, where English may not be their first language. So, it can quite hard sometimes to give them medical advice. I was just thinking in terms of the language barriers and sharing mindfulness practice, what is your opinion?

Devin – Yes, I think both. It will depend on the situation if you haven't got an interpreter; quite often you don't. You need be situational, breathing is universal, thinking is universal. If you just close your eyes, maybe the initial partnership is just to breath, that's a good start because this will settle down the nervous system and gradually, you can start to layer on different mindful practices depending on where they are. I mean a language barrier is certainly obtrusive, but it's not a deal breaker.

Arun – Finally, should mindfulness practice become mainstream as part of SP in pharmacies where patients are referred to mindfulness classes and practitioners to enable them to have a better control of their H&W? Mental health is becoming a growing problem and stress is almost an epidemic right now, in order to address that, should it become mainstream with every single pharmacy offering leaflets on mindfulness and a referral process?

Devin – In an ideal state or world, I think you should have a mindfulness room or an opportunity for patients to do it in the pharmacy. If you were prescribing something for wellbeing, it would be much easier for me to do it right there in a room or even go for a fifteen minute walk. When you prescribe medicines, why do you have to be behind the counter, what if we went for a walk for five or ten minutes, we talked so I get to exercise while we are engaging. There are so many things you could do change the situation, to contextualise it, make it more meaningful for the patient.

Arun – This is like 'Health Walk' where we have a group of people to walk together in a pre-planned path which increases social connections, and the walking path in a new environment helps improve their mental wellbeing substantially. Essentially, there have been some pharmacies offering it and the 2016 award winner for innovative projects organised by the RPS was a Health Walk Scheme. This goes a step closer for developing a stronger bond with the patient and going outside the box for enhancing their wellbeing.

Devin – You can have a meditation room, you can have a yoga room, there are so many little things you could do. I think you are in the pressing edge of changing the patient and pharmacist relationship, taking healthcare in the 21st century and make wellbeing one of the primary focus and I think mindfulness can certainly help you and others along that journey.

Interview with Billie Jordan from Hip Op-eration Crew

Billie – It was a mistake, you know. When I set them up, it was more just to give the elderly people something to do, but I didn't realise how big the impact would be on them. Now, we have lots of Hip Hop dance groups in New Zealand with senior citizens being set up and as you know, I am trying to set them up around the world because it creates so much improvement in their mental and physical health.

The key reason I think my dance group improves the health of so many of the senior citizens in the community is that there are many aspects of it. The exercise is probably the smallest bit. They are exercising without realising that. The big part of it is they are meeting other people and the good thing about dance is that it is not intellectual. You are meeting such a different group of people that you wouldn't otherwise meet, there are things which, usually, people have to have because they don't have to have dance experience, that's really important.

They are not meeting people who are just dancers, or like a book club which they usually use where you need people who are intellectually smart. This way, you are meeting people who are smart, and people who may not be; they are from different walks of life. So, it's the social aspect of meeting new people, but the other thing is that in my dance group, they all must do dance at the same time and that's really very crucial because it gives the sense of teamwork. They can't just act as one person, they must think as one team and that's healthy given we are social animals and being in a group is so important. So, they stop thinking about their own needs.

They think about the needs of everyone around them and they must move in their pace. They must know their person and moment details and what they may do to keep up, so they become very aware of other people around them. They need to do things as one group. The other thing that I think has worked for them so much is that I made them go to a competition. There are lots of exercise group for older people, but they don't enter them in any form of competition. It's crucial that the elderly have some representation in the game. They must have a risk factor and they have to have a threshold of performance and expectations of them, because otherwise it's patronising, and you don't get their brain working.

They need to be in competition to enter. I am not a competitive person and I have not have participated in team sport in my background, but I realise how crucial it is when you are an older person. The great benefit of that is if they get sick, you know they will have an injury or get sick because they are old, but the difference here is that they want to get out of bed quicker because they don't want to let the group down; the group are depending on them to perform well in the competition. I have one of my dancers who broke her pelvis – she is blind – but she was back dancing six weeks later because she didn't want to let down other people. She knew she was needed because everyone is to do the same dance in their spots. So, with one person out, everyone need to compensate for it, it's a hassle but that's the key.

This makes it detrimental to the group if one person doesn't turn up, it's crucial. So solely, they find themselves not needed by their family, by their children anymore but here they are needed. It's not a club where you just turn up when you want, they are needed. Other people suffer if they are not there. One of my dancers broke her leg but she was back up and dancing four weeks later.

Absolutely crucial, the thing I noticed with exercises, is balance, and they all have very good balance. I don't teach them balance but dance forces them to be on their legs so they have very good balance. The ratio of falls to the average population is very small. A lot of them will have disease, they may have a kidney problem, and I can't help them with that. Some of them have had heart attacks or strokes, one of them had a heart attack but that was 1 out of 80 people of my dancers. They just want to repair themselves quickly.

The competition is very crucial because there is an expectation put on them, they have to turn up because everyone is relying on them. They know their team will get a bad score if they are not there. So, the pressure is up, they know they are not going to win, I enter them in competitions and they will always come last but it's not the point. The good thing is they are out there and meeting young people who they are competing against. They have expectations upon them, they have pressure, they must care and think about each other, they have to be healthy and be there for each other. That is crucial.

There are too many places where the older generation have no expectations on them. I am not a dancer; I taught myself how to dance on YouTube. I just did it because I wanted older people to have a better of quality of life. I first got a teacher in, I had two dance teachers. So, each one, after the second one, I realised it was not going to work. I realised that I was going to have to teach them, because the first dance teacher had really low expectations of them, he was just like as long as you are having fun and moving, and I don't expect you to do well, and I thought that was demoralising.

The thing is, those who have the greatest obstacle in a group, especially a dance group, have the most to contribute because they inspire others. As a dance teacher, got rid of the professional dance teachers since I realised I am the only one who is going to be able to teach these people. I had two days to learn how to dance in popping, choreographer, routines and then start teaching them. I started learning how to teach people with dementia through basically trial and error.

The big thing was that by including people who have the most obstacles, the most major disabilities and who are the oldest, it sends a message to all the others that even if they struggle, I am not going to abandon them. A lot of older people have the feeling of being abandoned in their life from their family and friends, especially in the West, so that's important to me that they understand. I used to say even for the World Hip Hop Championship that you are going, even if you are in an urn or a coffin to give them certainty that, regardless of their mental or physical state, I am not going to abandon them. That way, they could feel that we are one big family, that they were valued that we weren't going to be abandoning them if they could not keep up with the team; it's not about the dancing at all, it's just an excuse.

The exercise, of course, is great, but there lots of places they could go to for that alone. So, I knew that's why I ensure I have so many old people who want to join, because they want to be somewhere where there are expectations of them, because they miss that. They had that when they were working and don't have that now. I give it back to them.

Arun – Thank you so much for sharing your story with me, I wasn't aware of this information from watching the videos, but now I have got it straight from you. I would like to add two things, one is Heart Intelligence. It's a company in America called Heart Labs, they did a study back in the 1980's and found that the heart gives out a frequency, and you can think of your body like an antenna; your heart is giving out electricity and it was found that the range is up to fifteen feet. You can receive the electric feedback from one heart to another and sentimentally when you said it's good to have all the people together, everybody is sending out good signals that they have the intention of taking part in the dance class.

It changes the biochemistry of the body to allow them to go further, and the other thing is sense of purpose. It was found that if somebody had any daily goals or any purpose even if its small, it could be like having a walk with the grandchildren, this enable them to live a longer life because they have something to wake up every morning, something to look forward to. Essentially, the observation that you have made is scientifically backed as well. Heart Intelligence fascinates me because that's why it's really important to surround yourself with positive people, they can send good vibes which refers to positive frequency from their heart, the magnetic field.

Billie – That's great to know; I noticed they really gelled together as soon as I put them in their first uniform. When we were wearing the same clothes for the first time, it changed – they were better dancers, they were happier group, they were more gelled – it was quite interesting to see the small changes just getting them in the same clothes. There is a 30 year age gap between the youngest and the oldest, you know. So, the good thing is even though the younger one had to go slower than perhaps they could, the upside for them is that they know that they won't be abandoned when they are older and in their nineties or become disabled.

They could see that they will still be included, even in later stages, they will still be given the green light ahead. It's interesting. The BBC did a story about my dance group from the medical benefits that they have. They interviewed the doctors on the island. Because we live on an island, it's a very controlled environment; we are all in the same environment. So, there was a group of old people that joined my group and a group of old people the same age on the island who didn't.

The BBC came and interviewed the doctors to see if you could tell a difference between those in the group and not in the group who lived in the same environment. They have seen that there was at least ten years younger in the ones who joined the group, their attitudes were positive, they required less medication than they did before, they recovered from any illnesses and injuries much quicker. They could tell even through the way they walked.

All the doctors in the island were interviewed for this study, and they were unanimous in observing the massive difference. In New Zealand, the highest age group of suicide is 65 and over because of depression and loneliness. The big thing with depression is their sense of purpose. The other thing which really lifted them was that they had never done hip hop dance before. Many older people will go to do an activity they have done before, and they will notice that they are not as good at it as they used to be. They will feel that with as they get older, that they are not as good at things they used to be. With Hip Hop dancing, there was no young self to compare themselves by – it was completely new to them – it wasn't like ballroom dancing which they did when they were younger. So, they could only find out that they were just getting better and better at something.

The other thing which I felt important was capturing them on social media, so I could send it to their grandchildren and their children, which then brought them into their lives because suddenly, that old person is relevant again. That is the benefit of hip hop; it is something younger people will do. This made them and all of a sudden, their grandchildren were interested in them again, where they weren't before.

It's so important that the elderly do what the younger generation are doing now, so that they can make better connections. A lot of elderly people will say *"I want to connect with young people, but it's got to be on my terms"*. The younger person must come and do the thing that I am interested in doing, the old person never goes and does what the young person is interested in doing. Start playing video games, learn how to skate board, learn how to hip hop dance, learn how to rap, do all of these things. Get on social media, have a blog; a blog by a 100-year-old will soon be watched by millions. Start doing the things that the younger generation do, so the elderly people must step up their game as well.

Arun – Have you heard of the term neuroplasticity? It's a concept that started over 100 years ago, but it was only scientifically proven in the 1970s. It's the ability of the brain to be plastic so that it can change in structure to accommodate new habits and new behaviours through the forming of new brain cells. Neuroplasticity is the ability of the brain to mould itself to learn a new skill. Neurogenesis is the ability of the brain to generate new neurons to install that new habit. What they did in a study was when a baby is born, throughout the first seven years of their life, the brain is 100 percent plastic. Anything they are learning in that time frame is very easy for them to pick up – it can be learning a new language, a new dance style or to play an instrument.

However, when you go past that seven year threshold, even from seven to twelve, for the brain to remain plastic, they have to learn something very interesting and it has to be a new skill. After the age of forty, the brain starts to decline in functions. One way to slow down the process, I wouldn't say reverse it but slow it down, is to learn a new activity. It could be learning a new language, it could be dancing, it could be doing brain health exercise online (BrainHQ). The reason you said that you noticed they were feeling happier and so on was that there was a modification done in their brain chemistry, because they are installing new habits of dancing. Like you said, they are getting better and better through the reward system, once they see an improvement, it releases dopamine, the feel-good chemical, which then makes the brain even more plastic.

Billie – That's very intriguing, as they will be looking at their dancing from a year ago and they will feel a little embarrassed because they are so much better now. It's a good thing. It's nice for them to have something that really keeps improving. I am really into any social activities that a person has never done before when they are older. I think that's very important to get the full effect.

Arun – Definitely, when you said skateboarding and rapping, I was surprised as I never thought of it but then after what you have accomplished, I can see it happening. If you have the vision, you can make it happen. That would be very interesting to see. Especially the 100-year old blog that would be getting millions of views, that's for sure.

Billie – Anything which young people are doing is what they should do, because otherwise they will become irrelevant. It's no different than if you know somebody dressed up like a medieval person, you know those who do sword play, who go to a corporation and saying this is how we will be beating our competitors; it's irrelevant. It doesn't work like that anymore, do you know what I mean? You beat your competitors through marketing and product enhancement, not through sword fighting, it does not work like that anymore.

To be relevant in society is not just to be valued as a person, but to be valued as a voice. They need to be relevant. More than ever, in the history of the planet, senior citizens have the largest voice they ever had; there will be more of them than young people in thirteen years' time. So, there is some huge weight but with that they would have more privilege.

I think older people need to because I have also noticed in my dance group because I am not immune from all personality types, so I have got people that no matter what I give them, present to them, they want to be treated like an invalid and infantile, like a child. Even though, they are physically fine. There is nothing wrong with them, so there is always going to be some people just based in their personality that's never going to accept or join any of those social activities. I think there is an important footnote that has to be, it's not the cure but there are some that no matter what I give them, free this, I will take them round a world trip, all expenses paid, everything, they will still turn it down because they would rather be viewed as an invalid and helpless, even if they are not.

That's just based on their personality and what I have noticed is that the one who were the youngest in my group, were more likely to be like that than the one who were in their eighties and nineties. This is because those in the 80's and 90's were clearly ill equipped to be Hip Hop dancers but they had a different attitudes or giving it go. The one in their sixties had better chance and were more physically able but there were still ones being there that were in the threshold of *"I will give it a go, but I would rather get a teaching through sympathy than in teaching to success"*. I will probably say that they would have been about 10 percent of my dance group would rather be in that group within to get attention from somebody. The problem is, you know, for a lot of older people, if they are lonely, how do they get attention.

If their friends are dying, the family are not interested in them anymore because they have become irrelevant or boring, you know, you shouldn't be boring and if you're going to be boring, who is going to be around you. The only way to get attention is to go a doctor and say to the doctor *"Oh, I have got pain in here"*, send them to the pharmacy, give the pharmacist another thing to check about the dosage then they go back home. Then the medicine works, and they are like *"How am I going to get attention now? Oh, I will say it's this shoulder now"* then I will go to the doctor then to the pharmacist, do you know what I mean because how else are they going to get attention. There is always something that's going to happen like that, no matter what you give them, they are going to do it.

I speak around the country a lot, and people come to me saying, *"I have an elderly person in my life and I am trying to get them to get out of bed and to have a bit of life"*, I say to them, well, if you think they are depressed then that's a different issue, they need to see a doctor. Depression is not a normal part of ageing. If you don't think they are depressed and they don't have the signs of it, you just have to think of ways to engage with them. If this still doesn't work, give up. Don't even waste your energy on them because I have wasted years on certain people to try to get them out, and it was pointless; this meant I had less energy to give to other people.

Arun – I completely agree with you. On a daily basis, as a pharmacist, sometimes I do see patients where I have a consultation, and the first two minutes would be about medicine, but for the remaining ten to fifteen minutes – the longest was 45 minutes – was just them talking about their personal life. I can relate on where they are coming from. They are always grateful for me listening to them afterwards, and I would say that it's my pleasure. I can relate to what you said, and I personally feel that some people once they reach a certain threshold, it's hard for them to change the brain chemistry because they always do the same thing.

Like you said, with the analogy of the crashing plane, you must put the oxygen mask on yourself first before putting it on the child. This is because if you don't help yourself first, you won't be able to help others. You tried your best already. You must focus your attention on those who may benefit from it more. So, you've done the right thing. It's the way of life, some people are tuned for positivity and some people are tuned for negativity.

Billie – The biggest mistake I made when I set up the group was that I did not charge for my lessons; it's all voluntary so I don't get paid. This was a big mistake because a lot of people like myself, like to give to others. It's usually because we have been through something ourselves so we sympathise. So, when I started the group, for the first three years, I came from an abusive background, so I had a low self-esteem and I felt like I was worthless as a person. I don't think that now. So, I just gave, gave and gave to almost earn my right to live, you know.

I had to show that I was worthwhile to breathe oxygen. I didn't have the self-esteem that I could have, that I am born and therefore I have a right to breathe oxygen. I thought I had to earn it. So, I sent a message that I was basically a doormat. By not charging, it reinforced it. I had a lot of my time and energy taken out with people who just like to have a doormat in their life and they took as much of my energy and time that they could possibly take from me.

I also had people in the group who were not there to be part of the group, but just there because they were bored and were kicked out of the other group. This is the only group which had no membership fee, there were no auditions, there was nothing to get through to get in the group. I was in Waikehe island where it attracts people who are in the fringe of society, they don't want to live in a mainstream thing, they want to live on an island, so Waikehe island is full of eccentric people who are not really conformers, I suppose. I had a miserable time with lots of people but then I grew my self-esteem slowly and my sense of worth.

I should have charged something because they needed to see value in what I was providing, and they don't unless you charge them. Even it was only two dollars, I should have charged them. I don't charge them now, but I only focus now on seven great people with great attitudes, the others I don't put my energy into. So, I think they need to have a stake in their own accord, like an investment financially, for them to value it because a lot of social services for old people are done by volunteers like me, so there must be, for it to be sustainable for the volunteers.

The volunteers must find it enjoyable and must have a certain amount of protection, or a certain amount of respect for them to be able to continue providing their service. There needs to be some sense of goodwill. Probably 60% of my dancers have never said thank you, ever, because of this. If I charge them, they will be, they are more grateful for the smallest things. After the World Hip Hop Championship, none of them said thank you. I met a lot of people who are volunteers in the senior citizens sector around New Zealand and a lot of volunteers do get treated like unfairly.

A lot of them have got experience of being treated badly because they are providing something for free. Their time is not seen as valuable, so I gave up my full-time work to just do this for those people. I paid $3,000 for one of them to get to Las Vegas and she never said thank you. I sold my possessions for that. So, I have learnt to hold back.

I didn't have any self-worth, I just wanted to give, and people just wanted to take. With my dance academy, in it, people train to be a dance teacher, I have a section there making all the dancers sign a sheet to abide by certain behaviours that are expected of them and, that they can be kicked out if they don't adhere to it. They also need to charge. It doesn't matter what it is, you've got to charge something. I tried to pass on what I learned, but I don't talk about all those negative aspects publicly because I know that I can bring much more good globally and inspire more people and if they continue to see what Hip Hop-eration do. I don't want anyone feeling bitter towards them, even some of them are inappropriate.

Arun – I can relate to your experience. For the first four years of me doing Krump, I have been based in UK. I would not get any productive feedback from any of my peers. I don't know if it's a cultural thing, but it was only when I started to travel that I truly felt part of a community. When I went to India in March 2014, prior to that I was teaching a few people on Skype, so I wanted to meet them personally. One of my students organised a workshop and it was very successful, and this is when I made the decision to use my wages as a pharmacist to bring my friends from across the world to come and teach in India.

I must have spent over £12,000 with my own money for the Indian krumpers to increase better knowledge and skills. In 2016, we had an Indian representative come to the World Championship of Krump and that was my ambition achieved. This is when I was able to make the decision to focus on myself, stop giving and giving so that I can write my book. I noticed since I started to invest money on myself doing courses, attending events, I feel so much more productive, and also, the seed I planted in India has grown into a very strong tree. There are four Indian krumpers going to Russia with a visa approved for competing at an event in July 2017, this is such a huge inspiration for me because I started with them from the very beginning.

Likewise, you have planted a seed which has become a very strong tree for the future generation and yourself. Any past experiences I know I could have done in different ways, but I have no regrets. A mistake becomes one only if done twice; I have learnt from it. I have become so much stronger as a result, it may be the same for you too. You are passing on your knowledge to any upcoming academy instructors. Essentially, it's your way of learning and its good people are getting involved with your academy.

Billie – It's true, I have learned about boundaries and valuing myself which I wouldn't have otherwise learned if I had not have been treated so badly. That's OK, I can help others to not fall into the same pit I did. I am excited, when I get old, I am going to learn how to be a stunt car driver, I am going to learn lots of things that I am not learning now. Different things, including travelling independently, that's one of the big thing for me to do.

Arun – In UK, the health sector tends to be separated from the arts sector. Through Social Prescribing (SP), it already happened in small cities where SP is being funded by the health care system in our country. My question is, have you thought to do a partnership with the department of healthcare in New Zealand to provide funding for the instructors? Because, essentially, what you are doing is a huge Social Return Of Investment (SROI). By making the dancer's health and wellbeing improve, you reduce the risk of fractures or falls which have a huge cost for the health care system in general. In the UK, it costs the NHS around £3,000 for a hip fracture. I strongly believe you should try to form a partnership and include the term SP because you already have all the evidence to help scale it as part of GPs, pharmacies, and care homes under the banner of Hip Hop-eration.

Billie – In New Zealand, there is no funding for anything to do with the elderly. If you were to set up something for senior citizens, you wouldn't be able to receive funding. But, the government here are doing a falls prevention program. They worked out that falls are costing the government a lot of money, and they used my Hip Hop-eration crew to make the leaflet to promote this initiative. But, it is not as simple as just telling somebody not to fall over; no-one wants to fall over. What will a brochure do? All they have done in New Zealand is make brochures telling people they should not fall over, because it is too costly.

Arun – This will increase the number of falls as they have become more consciously aware of it.

Billie – Yes, you are right, I should put more time into my dance academy because I have put no time into it. This should be provided to every senior citizens in New Zealand as standard. They do realise the benefits of it, they can see it. I had the people lead up the fall prevention program in New Zealand, and the government came to one of my rehearsal so that they could see it for themselves. It was tangible evidence, when I started playing the music they were just blown away, they couldn't believe these were a group of elderly people; they instantly got it. I don't have to write an essay about it because the evidence is there in the performance. They can see the faces, the joy and the comradely they are making.

They are physically doing things that they have never seen an old person being able to do. So yes, I would like to get young people, a franchised youth, becoming dance instructors. Train them to teach those old people, I want to do it through the youth system, but I need to focus on getting my head together.

Arun – The term you can use is value-based care. 75% of insurance is making payments using it. That means when a patient receives treatment, they get an initial payment. But, then after 90 days, if the patient doesn't improve, they receive a penalty fee, or they don't get any payment at all. If the patient improves, this is when they get a further payment. One of the pioneers is Kaiser Permanente who started in the 1950s and is known globally. The UK is trying to follow the same journey with Patient Activation Measures (PAM) scores which looks at patient empowerment for healthy lifestyles. In the USA, they use Accountable Care Organisations (ACOs) whereas in UK, they use Vanguards. There might be a similar organisation in New Zealand which focuses on value-based care. If there is, they would be the best partnership for your project once it scales up.

Interview with Julie from Move It or Lose It

Arun – What inspired you to start your company in improving the wellness of senior citizens?

Julie – At the time, I was a teacher in school and getting very disillusioned with the education system. My parents were elderly and started to suffer with health problems. I really wanted to do something which was going to be more rewarding and to also help me cope with my parents and what they were going through at the time. I did a training course chair-based exercises for older adults and then I went on to do further qualifications and exercise to music.

I started to deliver some classes and found that I loved doing it. It was the best job I had ever done. It was so rewarding and the people I was teaching were having such fantastic benefits and changes in their life due to the classes. It just made me think I've got to throw myself in and give this 100 percent. I thought wouldn't it be fantastic if this could reach not just the people in my class but thousands more, so they could the enjoy the same benefits. I began expanding on my classes and I was teaching more and more people – I could not keep up with the demand.

At that point my class members kept saying to me, *"We want to exercise more than once a week but cannot remember what to do when we go home"*. So, we tried all number of things to give them a reminder, but none were successful, so I ended up working with a film producer to make a good quality exercise DVD. The people in my class starred in it and they came up with the name "Move It or Lose It". I knew it would appeal to the same kind of people that were attending my classes, those who needed a chair-based exercise routine that they could then do at home. That's how it began.

From there, I met Professor Janet Lord, Director of the Centre for Healthy Ageing Research at the University of Birmingham and she encouraged me to make more DVDs to include weight-bearing and resistance exercises which we know, of course, are vital. Move it or Lose it became collaborating partners with the Centre, looking at the research and then translating it into practical and effective ways of getting people to move more. So, I continued and made five award-winning DVDs and then wrote a book.

During that time, I recognised that I couldn't really have as much impact if it was just me and the best thing I could do, would be to train people to deliver Move it or Lose it classes. This would mean that older people across the country would be able to come along to a safe, effective and enjoyable class where they could exercise and socialise.

So that's when we began the instructor training course and I developed the FABS course which includes flexibility, aerobics, balance and strength in the same class and can be done seated or standing. Our aim is to now train a thousand specialist instructors so that they can deliver Move it or Lose it! classes which also focus on the social aspect as well the exercises. People who would not normally exercise can come together in their local community to enjoy the group sessions and benefits that come from getting stronger, more mobile, improving their balance and confidence.

Arun – If the collaboration between your company and community pharmacy was to go ahead, would you have a FABS accredited instructor come personally to the pharmacy on a specific day to share the "Cuppa Routine" with the patients on a 1-to-1 or 1-to-many basis? The patients could be identified by staff members who think will benefit from this five minutes routine and most of the patients do have tea in the morning. This will reduce the risk of falls as their balance and core strength will be improved.

Julie – I think that would be fantastic because getting this in front of people is a difficult thing to do. The professionals that have regular contact with older people, could really make every contact count, and use that opportunity to guide them to do something in their own home that takes a couple of minutes yet can have a real impact.

We spoke to a lot of our class members and they say that they make about six cups of tea a day. So, I thought – what a great opportunity, they are in the kitchen, waiting for the kettle to boil, they could do some simple exercises and the act of switching on the kettle could be the regular prompt they need. Ultimately it becomes like Pavlov's dogs, so they think, *"I am putting the kettle on. Ding, that's my reminder"* to do my exercises. By the end of the day, they might have done 30, 40, 50 or even 60 sits to stands which they would never have done otherwise.

I think the 'prompt' is very important. We train our instructors to encourage their class members to be active every day at home, after each class we give them a little task to do in the week. It's almost like setting homework and saying to people *"Now this week, I want you to focus on doing the sit-to-stand or trying to improve your balance with the heel-raise or doing your pelvic floor exercises"*. It needs to be made easy and accessible so that's why the cuppa routine work very well and if there was something we could do with pharmacies to promote that, then it would be fantastic.

Arun – You could collaborate with CPPE to develop a training course for pharmacies to become familiar with the FABS course content, including the cuppa routine. This can go towards our CPD portfolio to help us meet the NHS 5YFV objectives.

Julie – That would be perfect because then everybody is aware, we all need to take some responsibility for health promotion whether it's family, doctors, pharmacists, exercise instructors or nurses. We can all do something to promote activity and healthy living. It's a gentle way of encouraging rather than to threaten which sometimes comes over in typical health messages. Getting someone to go from no activity to a little activity still has an impact. Just like the app that's been released from Public Health England (PHE), "Active 10" which aims to get people to walk briskly for ten minutes every day.

A lot of people we teach would not manage walking for ten minutes at a brisk pace, but after doing our classes they can improve their balance, strength and confidence and then become more active in everyday life.

Arun – You also have your dedicated app "Move It or Lose It" to assist participants to track their progress.

Julie – Yes, we now need to develop the app to send out video content to help people exercise in their home, prompt and remind them to attend classes and track their progress. We need more funding to go to the next stage but that's on the card.

Arun – Could you tell me more about the FABS course?

Julie – Yes, all the theory is done online before attending the two-day practical course. In advance they watch videos of every exercise and how to relate these to activities of everyday living. Then during the practical sessions, they are assessed on their ability to deliver the programme safely and effectively.

Arun – Is it open to anybody, like occupational therapists and dance instructors?

Julie – Yes, there are two courses, the "Fast Track" for people who have got an existing fitness qualification at level two or above and they do a shorter online course. Then the "Full Course" is for people who haven't got any previous experience or qualifications and they have a longer online course. We have found that people who have come in with no previous qualifications often turn out to be fantastic instructors, particularly those in their fifties or sixties who are doing this because they don't want to retire completely but they want to do something rewarding and give something back. The main thing is for instructors to have empathy and motivational skills which are just as important as having knowledge.

Arun – Have you considered undergoing a partnership?

Julie – Yes, we have officially partnered with Royal Voluntary Service, they have 35,000 volunteers all over the country. Their volunteers can help the people that they go and visit to do some simple exercises at home and then encourage them to come along to a local class for fun and company too.

We are seeking funding to help us expand this approach, so we can help thousands more people across the country.

Arun – Sweatcoin are a technology company who reward patients for walking and they are working with the Institute of Digital Healthcare based at the University of Warwick. You could collaborate with them for rewarding participants in digital currency.

Julie – That would be amazing because everybody likes an incentive and reward. We were thinking with our app that we could get people to receive bronze, silver and gold rewards. If somebody is already doing something similar, it might be easier to tie in with them using their tech platform. Maybe we could then offer to provide some video content and trial it – that sounds exciting.

Interview with Lady Christine Bamford from CID London

Arun – In your opinion, does the art sector tend to be isolated from the health sector? In that regard, what are your thoughts on a collaboration between GPs and dance practitioners/ organisations to run a scheme for people who are socially isolated? Especially those who are over 60 or may be suffering from a neurological condition like Parkinson's and MS, as it breaks down social isolation. Also, the essence of dance is joy with the music. Making a partnership more prominent between the health and dance sector.

Christine – This is based on my experience, I worked in health for 20 years. I am a great supporter of health and wellbeing through dance and movement as president of CID UNESCO. I worked with GPs, medical practitioners and my feeling is that it's gathering momentum. There is an understanding with having the sort of tag as social prescribing. There is a greater understanding by GPs that there is a need for something else other than prescribing drugs. So, I particularly like your tag-line about Movement Pharmacy. There is quite lots of research going on that I think you can utilise and a number of people who are now starting to create a movement where actually not just dancing but the arts in general can be used in a therapeutic way.

I would like to recommend you also to contact with the dance and creative wellness network. I will connect you to those because there are people mainly in Europe who are using movement to mainly people with Parkinson's and MS. So, I think it's useful for you to look at that model and Julie Robinson from Move It Or Lose It, look at her website, she is just doing what I would call straight forward movement for the over sixties. I think she brings some sort of measurements.

In the medical profession, because it's so generated by lots of people with lots of different brains, there is always not a political interest in whatever happens, so whatever you may spend your money on, you have to be able to withstand scrutiny of it. So, you don't want to end up in front of a newspapers. It's quite useful if you can show to GPs and associate prescribers what impact it has, like Movement Pharmacy, is making and measured difference in health outcomes. So, I think it's useful if you wish to explore further, you could have qualitative measures like '*I feel fab*', '*I feel better*', '*I feel less isolated*' but how you would show the impact via different measures. I would encourage you to explore that more fully but be prepared if you are making an offering to the CCGs or to GPs. You can give them some sort of measurements if they purchase many sessions for people who have a medical condition, you know like how would you help them know that you've made a difference to them.

Arun – I tried to run dance classes for people who are socially isolated in Swindon, so I had a meeting with somebody from the Social Prescribing Team back in January 2017. However, for some reasons, it fell through despite several attempts to follow up. I will be aiming to start classes in Stroud and I will get in contact with the local Parkinson's group. Also, to potentially convince the CCG to make it formalised and possibly try to inspire more pharmacy schemes related to dance across UK. That's my ambition.

Christine – Have a look at some of the videos with people with Parkinson and the differences it makes when they start to move. See if you could capture that if you are going to have discussion with CCGs or your LPC. Nailsworth is a very small town and the GPs in the Stroud area are quite progressive. If you can go with the right sort of information and evidence because there is quite a lot of evidence on the differences movement can make to Parkinson. Then, you can ask for a deferred payment because money is there to be spent. If you can show that you can make a difference and if you have Parkinson in that area, it's quite difficult to get anywhere without transport which may be an issue. They will work better in a small area. Gather your evidence because there is a lot out there and then go and see them. You also need to see if you can find the percentage of the population across Gloucestershire area that may have Parkinson's or MS because there is a sort of similar degenerative condition.

When I was in Berlin, we had a movement workshop under the dance and creative network. We had people who came in with Parkinson's and MS. It's astonishing that after a while, you could not tell notwho was able-bodied and who was not. That was within 10 to 15 minutes. So, you know, you could put a one-off to show and that can be very powerful. You can involve the charity people, they can then influence the GP or the CCGs. You can do videos on what's' about or interviews about the difference it made. So, you can then present that people who may fund it. It's so astonishing if you can show a clip before and get some feedback from the individuals.

There were two things that were face striking, one it was Parkinson and MS sufferers, so what they valued was us being in a class not just with people who have a condition but others because it made them feel more normal. Just having that opportunity and that space, you know the shake and all the conditions disappear and what differences it made just for that moment in time. It's a very powerful stuff if you capture it, use stuff from YouTube, use your own but show what a difference it made locally.

With Silver Swans, there is a big movement coming about movement and dance because with dance, you have choreography which affects cognitively. It is made to people with long term conditions and staying healthy and well. This also reduce isolation, there is a big movement and her show (Angela Rippon CBE) was part of promoting that. She got new BBC documentary coming out later this year.

Arun – There are public health campaigns done with pharmacists like smoking cessation, alcohol consumption, sexual health and flu awareness. As a dancer, I would love to see a collaboration for a dance campaign. In your opinion, what would be the necessary steps of making it happen, will it be best to approach yourself as CID President for a campaign kit. This can then be used to bring it to the attention of pharmacy managers for promotions of physical activity.

Christine – Yes, we could do that. We can also do a collaboration with dance and creative wellness network in Berlin. They do something around November so that would be quite useful. Let's see how we can do that. I think it would be quite useful to approach some of the big pharmacy network and see if there is an appetite for promoting it.

Arun – At the HLP Training Event, it is an initiative for pharmacies to do more services around health and wellbeing. One of the key points was to offer new services, this is what made me think of dance where most pharmacies will become HLP. Promoting dance for HLP will be the best option for making it happen.

Christine – That would be a good idea where there is a shift to take some of the pressures off GPs to stop chronic conditions by reducing GP visits.

Arun – What's your opinion on having a dance programme for care homes? There was a study done which found out the residents can be malnourished. I am sure they don't do physical activity because they tend to be quite limited on what they can do. What would be your opinion on running a pilot for dance classes in care homes, to make the residents more physically active though dance?

Christine – There are progressive care homes where there are many dance practitioners who are already doing that. Gail Borrows is one of them. There is not a sort of global movement but it's always quite useful to approach chains of care homes. Like what we have here in Bristol, they are a quite respected establishment and they do all sort of activities. I don't know if they do movement as such but certainly it's a useful thing. There is lots of community groups, there is no doubt you can put movement into some of the communities' centres. It does make a difference but then again, there is no one I know who is doing it at whole scale if you like but it's a really good idea. You can also do seated exercises.

Arun – We do have patients with cancer coming to our pharmacy at a stage it can be controlled with the medication, like Tamoxifen. What are your thoughts on having people with cancer attending dance classes? To help them take their mind off their condition?

Christine – Yes, you can flag them under like 85% of all chronic diseases are lifestyle induced and that include some cancers. So, cancer and movement can be part of the prevention agenda, but you can also be part on helping in early stage along with medication and other stuff. I think it's quite useful to look and see what research has been done on supporting cancer and mobility. This is because it's all part of the lifestyle and quality on improvements in a whole range of stuff. You could also be starting to offer if you have anyone connected to nutrition because there are a number of things to make a difference to health and wellbeing like dance movement.

The sole creativity which is very hard to move connects your soul to isolation, we ticked that box. There is also nutrition and there is also sleep that are key factors in maintaining health and wellbeing. So, it's quite useful for you maybe to be able to if there are any fact-sheet or anything which may be of interest like videos to be able to start offering health and wellbeing handouts which can be part of your pharmacy. This is because it is part of the body and part of the cognitive ability but also what can help you either stop prevention or start to maintain a special quality of life right up to end stage. That would fit neatly under the pharmacy umbrella.

That's the direction of travel, you could work with pharmacist and some of the GPs has rooms. You could be running teaching events and movement where you can bring somebody along to talk about nutrition. You could offer a whole wellbeing package which movement is a key point essential to that.

Interview with Chris Stenton from Community Dance

Arun – Should dance classes be offered to all patients identified as socially isolated or lonely as part of Social Prescribing (SP) in a pharmacy setting?

Chris – Yes, absolutely. Actually, one of the principles of participatory dance is about removing barriers to participation, and that includes responding to peoples' needs when they find themselves in socially isolated situations. This, for me, is part of the process of inclusion as well as access. It's about the language that you use, the strategies you put in place to engage people, how you talk to people, where you hold stuff; looking at some of the other very practical barriers that might affect say isolated older adults like transport or feeling welcomed to a building. The kind of barriers that might prevent people engaging with arts activities more generally are well-documented.

Social prescribing within a pharmacy isn't something I am familiar with unlike via a GP or practice nurse. I kind of understand how it works but I've never heard of it in a pharmacy setting.

Arun – Yes, currently it's not being fully utilised, and I am trying to increase the awareness with this book to make referral services available across all the pharmacies in UK in addition of GPs and nurses. This is to help identify patients who are socially isolated who may not appear to be the case when they visit the doctor, but it can be quite apparent to the pharmacist when they have a fifteen minutes conversation about their medications. Many people tend to open up, so that's when I saw they will definitely benefit from it.

Chris – Now, I understand more clearly what you are driving at. In which case then, it's probably a question about the kind of information that pharmacist has access to, about the kinds opportunities out there that they think may be appropriate for the person they are consulting.

There may be some kind of barriers around the perception of dance, which I think do exist in certain parts of the medical profession. They may have a very fixed view of what dance means and who can dance. It can be quite a challenging concept and there might be some risks associated with, for example, physical activity for someone who has a particular condition or set of conditions or lifestyle challenge, or whatever. So, fixed views on what dance means might impact on whether they feel it is an activity they are able to recommend.

Arun – Now that you have said it, something just came to mind: because you offer so many courses, have you considered to offer a course specifically for healthcare professionals (HCPs)?

Chris – I would love for us to offer this, and I may consider it. Great idea.

Arun – Because it came to my mind, if you had that course, you could give a certificate to say that person has got the correct knowledge to refer patients to dance classes, similar to what we have for Dance for PD. I also did the Safe Into Practice pilot back in February 2017, that's some of the ways we could break down the barriers and perception. For example, we did parkour today, what was in my mind was jumping around building, I may break a bone but after doing the course with the gentlemen, he broke it down to make it inclusive for everybody, it was just a magical experience.

Chris – Well, exactly, that's one of the things that is great about dance because it's really good in reaching out and engaging with people who are excluded from other activities.

I guess for me its people having the information that they need to decide about whether to 'prescribe' or not. I know that it exists in some areas of the NHS – some GP surgeries for example – and I know of some examples of a 'social prescribing directory' to help with prescribing activities and referring people on. There is a role for providing examples in leaflets, and that kind of thing. My understanding of some of the early progress in the sphere of dance for health and wellbeing is of the impact of some individual trailblazers who had a belief on what dance could do. What you're talking about is still quite new, for some people, so perhaps some kind of signposting tool made for the medical profession about patient engagement with arts opportunities could work well.

Arun – By any chance, have you seen the documentary "How To Stay Young" with Angela Rippon OBE, I believe. She was a presenter.

Chris – Yes, I have seen some of it.

Arun – Then she went to Germany and there was a pilot study between two groups over six months, one for cycling and the other dancing. The result was that dance provided much higher results and positive outcomes.

Chris – Absolutely and associated outcomes which are to do with the social activities and aspects of dancing. It's about being part of community. It can be really hard to answer questions about the 'other things dancing does' because a lot of the noise around dance, health and wellbeing is often about physical activity or inactivity. And yes of course, dance is a physical activity; you move, you are exercising; but it's a lot more than that. The 'value added' aspect of dance is the creative part plus exercise plus a sense of community and interacting with other human beings. This can be difficult to pin down and describe the impact of (than say, calorie burn or exercising to become out of breath) – but these 'softer' outcomes are really important outcomes.

Actually, it's perfectly possible to exercise and raise your heart without engaging with others within a group, and in most cases with dance you are in a group, so that helps with this issue of isolation.

Arun – Yes, from the statistics, I don't know how it was validated but it said that people who are socially isolated have a fifty percent increased risk of developing coronary heart conditions which is a very worrying figure.

Chris – Well, connectedness touch and human contact—is one of the very basic thing we need as human beings. Dance can be about this, engaging with others in the process of art making and moving together in whatever way is right for them. Dance is, of course, a physical activity but I would argue that we need to place the creative, social, and human interactive aspects of dance in the foreground.

And that actually requires people to champion it, in this way. In some of the early developments of dance in health contexts, some health professionals said, *"I really notice that when some of my patients engage with dance, this other really good stuff happens"*. It doesn't just improve their physical fitness, it has lots of other positive outcomes. That was at a time when it was unusual to talk explicitly about dance in a health context. Those people were trailblazers, and you need them. There are some trailblazers currently championing dance for people living with specific conditions. I can really sense a drive for pharmacies being used far more fully for healthcare and wellbeing and imagine the same kind of thing would be true in kind of Social Prescribing via pharmacies, because it's not really the first thing that you think of.

Arun – Yes, there was a document published in 2014 called the NHS Five Year Forward View (5YFV) which was tackling the issue that we need to go from a reactive approach to a proactive approach as they wanted to merge the gap between health and wellbeing. So, there has been an increased shift for pharmacies to become HLP accredited which means Healthy Living Pharmacy. It includes everyday physical activity and dance can be promoted as part of the campaign.

Chris – Public Health England's physical activity strategy, Everybody Active Everyday, shows that dance has a role to play, but I get I am nervous that the value-added benefits of dance are getting lost within the physical activity agenda. We need somehow to make sure that pharmacists and pharmacies have the right kind of information to signpost people to the right kinds of dance opportunities.

It's very much about context, about having the right kind of information from sources you can trust. Nobody wants to be signposting people to stuff which may not be good. But it's not just a one-sided responsibility. People providing the information to patients need to ensure they have the right kind of information and knowledge to pass on.

Arun – With the emergence of wearable trackers and the Internet of Things (IoT), should a pilot be carried out to provide quantitative results (e.g. health parameters) rather qualitative results (e.g. interviews)?

Chris – That's an interesting question, and I would have thought it is happening in some places already. I am not aware of a dance initiative which does exactly what you have described with using wearable pedometer or whatever, but I am pretty sure people are beginning to utilise technology to kind of, for example, work out quite literally the distance you travel by moving in a dance class.

Arun – When we measure people's outcome, we tend to do it maybe at the end of the class, maybe after two weeks or in a weekly basis, you have one measurement. However, by having a continual measurement 24/7, we can see the peak and the dip. This gives a broader picture on the overall benefit of rather than just a snapshot. So, having more data, and if interpreted correctly, can have a much more powerful case to the health sector and the NHS to embrace dancing.

Chris – Again, really interesting. I would imagine people would contribute to gaining that knowledge as say, wearing FitBit 24 hours a day for five weeks, that is no big deal really. And if it helps provide the data and I am sure people would be happy to do that.

Arun – They can also just wear it during the class.

Chris – Yes, so you could begin to capture exactly what happens in the room literally with the health parameters you talked about. So, describing the journey becomes a useful tool for people when recommending a particular activity as a good thing.

Arun – Definitely, because one of the latest developments is some people may be able to develop a device that can measure brain waves accurately. So, whenever somebody does a dance class as part of a group, the brain release dopamine, the feel-good chemical, to show how relaxed they are. There could be a pilot with a controlled group where after six weeks of dance classes and people over 60 who do absolutely nothing, we can show the brain waves in comparison to people who didn't showing a much higher level of relaxation. That could be an additional parameter which we could use to talk about the creativity in some way.

Chris – Yes, there are a few research-based projects which included control sample groups and these were able to set out some very interesting findings. There seems to be lots more research being done. Wouldn't it be interesting to know not just how physically active you've been, but have you become happier? Are you smiling more? Are you talking more? Are you interacting with people differently? There are things that can happen when you dance, and perhaps for longer as a result of dancing. It would be interesting to know whether there is IoT that would help measure that.

Arun – Now that you mentioned it, which connected the dots for me, I watched a video this morning about a device connected to the jacket of workers in a construction site. It measured how many times they go down and whether the posture of the back and bending are done correctly, and it shows up in the system. There is also a AI that can identify whether a person is happy or sad, in terms of design, I haven't figured out yet, for example, let's say we had the participant wear a headband with an attached camera which can see the facial expression and identify how the changes occur. The design needs to be improved but that's just an idea.

Chris – This stuff is becoming much more possible. If we can utilise technology to provide some hard and soft data alongside people actually talking about how they feel as a result of dance, then that would be a strong position to be in.

Evidence suggests that dance has been able to get a foothold in some spheres of health and wellbeing. I'm convinced this is because people have experienced it and believe in it, with some very strong champions and advocates. But even this can still be fairly localised. There might be a collection of health professionals who are very comfortable with this stuff and there will be others who just aren't. I am really interested in the opportunity of introducing pharmacies to dance. It's another layer that people interface with – you said 1.6 million people visit pharmacies each day, that's a lot of people and in terms of information provision, it feels like something we all need to address.

Arun – The advantage is from the ability to walk in a pharmacy and speak to a pharmacist with no appointment needed. Whereas for GP, it may take a few days to see one from booking an appointment.

Chris – There always seem to be queues in pharmacies, so you know a lot of people are using them! I think that's a really interesting proposition. The role of the HCP in this is key. I am interested in turning health professional into dancers, not dance artists in to healthcare professionals.

There is a job to be done of building bridges between people with ideas and concepts of health and wellbeing, but allowing people to be really good at what they do. For me, it's about being comfortable around ambiguity and some of those softer outcomes, like I know people smile more, that they connect together and that's alright. On one level, I don't need to understand any more than that, we can see what is happening.

Arun – Yes, having a good health is one thing but living a better quality of life (QoL) like smiling is much more important.

Chris –That's precisely it and I guess literately everybody has a role to play in that. Dance can have a role in enabling people to live well.

Arun – There is no language barriers as well, and that's the beauty of it.

Chris – Yes, many of the physical barriers can be counted as well which help make it inclusive. Like seated dance for example. It's a way of enabling people to participate and feel engaged, and as a result might be moving or interacting or communicating in a different way, or just at all.

Arun – Yes, I was able to signpost a patient to Swindon Dance for PD class and I changed his perception when I said that the class is done seated initially to warm up the muscles. He was really keen to take part after that.

Chris – In my understanding, and generally speaking, most people don't dance in order to be healthy, but they know that as a result of dancing, they are 'well'. I think the language is literally quite dissatisfactory around all of this because it's difficult to find the right kind of words to describe what we mean or feel. Saying "when I dance, I feel better" is not the same as saying "I go dancing in order to be healthy". In more nuanced than that, though the latter might be true too.

Thinking about your questions about the IoT if it's possible for marketing people to track our shopping habits in supermarkets – down to which shelf we look at first, and the face we pull at the price or label – then why not think about this in terms of dance? It must be possible to use this technology for good works! But I can't underline enough the importance of talking to people about their experiences too.

Arun – By having a specific goal, such as a performance at the end of 3 months. could motivate senior citizens to engage in dance classes (e.g. Hip Hop-eration performing at HHI), should all cities have a dedicated programme, dedicated to classes followed by a performance?

Chris – Performance and the motivation of and from this is important to people, even if that isn't the original motivation for participating. Whenever we talk to people about their community dance experience of being a participant and engaging with the others, people invariably talk about the importance of performing, sharing and showing their dancing. Very often, this is what most people are most nervous about particularly if they have never danced before. We did a piece of research in 2016 about older people dancing, which revealed the very interesting statistic that 85 percent of the activities led to performance or sharing.

There are perhaps issues here about confidence, identity as an individual and part of a group, building a new community, engaging with people if you are isolated. That's not necessarily what people set out to do, but something they discover. Taster activities can be very important. We still have lots of work to do about being able to show people what happens in a dance class, and what they can expect to experience as the result of taking part.

Helping people understand what their experience of engaging with dance might be is important. As is being able to provide the health care professionals with reassurance about quality, safe and responsible practice.

Arun – What should be the appropriate steps to engage with the STPs and CCGs to provide funding for Social Prescribing involving Dance classes?

Chris – Everybody is under immense pressure when it comes to money and resources.

Arun – One thing I would like to add is CCG have a Personal Health Budget (PHB) for some patients with a long-term condition (LTC) which is £96 per month I believe. This can be put towards activities that are going to improve their health outcomes. When I went to the Digital Health & Social Care Congress at the King's Fund, there was an organisation which helps patients make decision on how to spend their PHB as points via a mobile app.

Chris – I know of people who use their PHB to help them, for example, actually get to their dance group.

I guess in order to engage with CCGs more broadly, it goes back to the earlier discussion about information, champions and advocates. There is clearly a difference with the commissioning landscape for services which are about specific conditions and public health commissioning. Increasingly, I see less resistance in both fields. But I also see that there isn't enough money, and not enough time for people to do their work. Both factors can stifle the kinds of innovation we are talking about. Increasingly, though, with CCGs there are some good examples of where dance has worked very well and generates excellent outcomes for their users, both in terms of managing or preventing specific conditions and contributing to living well.

Arun – I mean someone who has a CHD cost the NHS money and social isolation increase the numbers of patients in that category. So, I think that's a strong case to look at when actually promoting wellbeing.

Chris – In some instances yes, but I have no interest in forcing people to do dance if they don't want to! In fact, it's absolutely fine not to; but it's not fine to be prevented from doing so. Dance should be there alongside other options. We just have to find a way of fitting together.

Arun – Have you heard of STPs, there are 44 of them governing 207 CCGs and 75 percent of them support SP.

Chris – Yes, I have heard of STPs. It would be interesting to know what they mean by 'supported'.

Arun – An improvement in health and wellbeing through dance can have a positive SROI, the NHS and NICE embraces RCTs to demonstrate evidence of efficacy, what would be the best methodology to meet the criteria?

Chris – I don't know what would be the best methodology, but my hunch is that it's not just one approach, but something that can meet a number of diverse needs and provide different levels and analysis of data. Facts and figures are essential, but so are peoples' voices.

Interview with Louisa Borg-Costanzi Potts from Trinity Laban

Arun – In your opinion, having a referral service from pharmacies to a dance practitioner would be ideal to speed up the uptake of dance classes for senior citizens, especially those over 65 as an example.

Louisa – Yes, from my perspective, the pharmacists/GP role is quite different here in the UK. Most of the time, older adults will visit their GP to get a referral to an activity which will support their health and wellbeing. I am not sure how this is different to what happens internationally. I do think if pharmacists or professionals working in the medical industry have referral information to signpost people to activities that would be very helpful. In my experience, it's the GP who has the 'weight' to more successfully encourage older adults who might be nervous about attending a dance class – potentially because they don't have any experience or/and their perception of what dance is makes them think dance isn't for them.

The GP is better placed to support the older adult to attend and to feel confident to do so but yes, I do think prescribing dance would be incredibly beneficial. The other thing to consider is the type of dance and the content of the 'offer'. GP's would need a lot more information about the activity itself, who/what the type of activity is useful for. It would need some way of being quality assured so in that respect, it would need more work from the delivering art organisation or from the health professional themselves to understand what it is that the activity is and needs to be, in order to be beneficial to people of all ages and abilities. Needless to say, there is some practice out there which is poor dance practice and could actually cause more harm than good to some participants and patients.

So, I think there is definitely something about quality assurance that has to be fed to that type of process. It would be very beneficial, but we would need to make sure that there are other things in place so that people are able to access the right high-quality activity for them.

Arun – Have you heard of "Dance for Health" by Tim Joss from AESOP? The pilot aim is to provide a framework to enable more dance practitioners to undergo the training for quality assurance, like you mentioned. There is also "Silver Swans" which is essentially ballet classes for senior citizens so rather than having several different projects across UK, do you think there should be one umbrella organisation which gathers all those different projects under one to enable to provide that quality framework for dance practitioner to teach seniors citizens.

Louisa – Yes, I have heard of both, and the answer is no, I don't. This is because there is a myriad of different approaches to delivering dance and reducing it down to one framework or one approach isn't going to work for everybody. Not every senior citizen is going to take part and enjoy the Dance for health program because it has a very particular approach. From what I know, it has physiotherapy exercises are included/embedded in the process. I haven't been to any classes myself, but I have attended conferences about it. So, I understand that this is a particular model and it works for some people but it's not a model which work for everybody.

For example, lots of our older adults that attend our classes here are at Trinity Laban wouldn't appreciate that particular approach. They don't like being associated with anything which assumes a medical intervention or that they need 'fixing/healing'. They much prefer a creative, artistic approach which actually gives them confidence, engages them, inspires them but still addresses potential mobility or cognitive issues as well as ensuring retention.

Since the older adults are enjoying themselves and of course they feel that they are being artistically challenged, they actually continue to come back to those classes and therefore we have fantastic attendance. Some of our older adults have been with us for five years and they have been coming every week because they are artistically and creatively engaged. Not necessary because they are thinking about whether they can touch their toes or any kind of physiological progression for them. Although, most will progress physiologically, but that isn't their main reason which brings them back. They feel better within themselves, they get the opportunity to meet other people, they feel more confident with their body but fundamentally, they feel like artists and that's why they keep coming.

So, I think there are many approaches which are suitable for lots of people because we are all different, so we can't do a one size fits all approach. It's not appropriate, it also disregards a lot of dance practices, some of them very good practice which has emerged from the community dance sector in the past fifty or sixty years which has huge impact on older adults and its very beneficial for them. This approach wouldn't fit within a more standardised medicalised model.

Arun – Have you heard of Hip Hop-eration crew? They are the world's oldest dance crew from New Zealand who participated at Hip Hop International (HHI) with the youngest being 66 years old and the oldest being 92 years old. They went to Las Vegas to compete in 2013 and they have a documentary and Hollywood movie being made about their story from Billie Jordan. What got me inspired when I first saw some of the clips last year was rather than just giving dance classes, they had a purpose, they knew after training, they would have to go and perform in front of a large audience in America.

Originally, they were socially isolated, put away from the society and having that goal is what enabled them to pursue it further and put more efforts behind it. So, in your opinion, should there be some kind of schemes so that when we do dance classes to enable to improve their creativity to actually have a goal for those interested to perform to an audience like a charity show or it could be an event locally. For example, Sadler's Wells have their Elixir festival which involves senior citizens. So, what is your opinion of having a combination of dance classes and for those interested to have a performance to break away from the stereotype that senior citizens cannot perform.

Louisa – I think performances are important to provide profile for a normally invisible group and publicly challenge issues relating to older adults/older bodies performing/dancing. Dancing in particular has a lot of challenges relating to aesthetics and performance and what a dancer's body should look like, how a dancer's body should move. The only way, we can start to challenge that notion is if we start to raise the profile and make visible another way of moving, another way of performing and more and different dance aesthetics. I think performance is usually important for lots of under-represented people including people with disabilities to be on stage and be seen, I think anything which can challenge a conventional notion of what dance looks like or who can dance is very important.

In terms of the offer for older adults, just as a sort of personal anecdote, I have been running the older adults program here at Trinity Laban for five years and it's been going for just longer than that, around six years. It's taken us about three years to get our participants to feel confident enough to want to perform. I think it's a really important thing to remember is that sometimes older participants (or any participant for that matter) who take part in dance aren't doing it necessarily because they want to perform. There could be a myriad of other reasons to take part – performance shouldn't be assumed. Co-design, coproduction and agency become really important anchor points of this type of work.

Although, despite not wanting to perform, our participants do want to go on an artistic journey, they want to be creative in a space of others and they want to develop those creative and artistic skills. However, that doesn't always necessarily mean they want to then present their work in a performative way or on a performance platform. I think that having that as a choice is really important. Of course, there are some participants that absolutely want to do that and having that option to be able to perform particularly as we are a performance art form, an expressive form.

I do think the offer should be there and we should try and push as much of it as possible but the option to not perform should also be there. So that people can feel the art form is accessible.

Arun – In terms of risk, so for example, when the GP or potentially the pharmacist refers a patient to a dance class and they agree to do it, would the accountability following an injury be associated with the dance practitioner or the GP or pharmacist for referring that person to dance class in the first place, in your opinion?

Louisa – For me, the responsibility always lies with the artist/ delivering organisation to adhere to best and safe dance practice, to be trained effectively, to be able to know how to deliver a dance class safely for participants with a range of needs. I think its important to have public liability so all artists who work in freelance capacity or within an organisation are covered, as accidents do happen particularly with dance as a physical art form.

So, I think the responsibility for the participants always rests with the dance artist/delivering organisation. It's up to them to ensure the delivery of a safe session. As well as ensuring they are trained effectively. I think it would be the responsibility of the GP or the health service in general if it does become something that we prescribe, to ensure the activity they prescribe meets their quality standard. So that's what I meant at the beginning about what are the quality principles that the GP will be looking for and what's the process to assess and understand where that quality is being upheld in those different classes/contexts.

Fundamentally, liability will always fall on the dance artist or the organisation delivering that session and it will always be their responsibility to ensure that they are well researched, well informed to be able to deliver a safe class for older adults who may have a myriad of different ailments.

Arun – In terms of the dance sector and the health sector, for the latter we have a budget set out by the NHS and then you have the arts sector funded by Arts Council England I think. In your opinion, who should be funding the program? Should it be a collaboration between the NHS and Arts Council England which is with the Big Lottery Fund or should it more like just the arts sector funding it, or should it be just the NHS?

Louisa – Well, we are in a complex funding landscape. I think in an ideal world, it's a combination but to be honest, I feel funding for this type of activity which crosses arts activity and Local Authority services should be financially supported by the local authority. So currently, at the moment, lots of the funding for our LA is being cut and removed which is diminishing the commissioning power that our LA used to have. The LA used to be able to commission health-related activities, some of those activities would be art-based but now that has been shifted and that responsibility lies with something called a CCG.

The issue with that is that group is made up of people who work in health as opposed to people who work in health and in the arts. Therefore, the arts activities tend not to really have much value within that context, potentially because members of the CCG may not be aware of the benefits the arts can have. So, I think it always need to be in combination but ideally, it comes from the LA who can ascertain where the needs are within the borough, it has a sort of breadth of understanding around the services which are out there including the arts service and the health services.

It also has that overarching view of the sort of companies and organisations that could work successfully in partnership. I do think that in a sense, the money should come from LA more than Arts Council or directly from the NHS. If that isn't possible then it depends on its nature, I think the NHS should be investing more money in arts interventions. I know that they are funding the arts on a small scale, but more work could be done to better integrate the arts into health and social care services, and this needs to come from the NHS/health professionals themselves.

The arts can do some incredible things in relation to engaging older adults isolated in their home for example. So, I do think more funding should be from the NHS, ideally a combination that is funnelled through the LA who have the local expertise. They can see where it should go and know who will provide quality activity. They have that knowledge much better than the NHS who are further removed from the locality.

Arun – Have you heard of STPs before (Sustainability & Transformation Partnerships)? You know you have the CCG which is essentially clinical commissioning group. I completely agree with you, it's made up of doctors and HCP. Similarly, to you guys as dancers, even pharmacists feel secluded. Essentially any service that aims to extend the level of service, who come to pharmacies, is restricted by people present in CCG. However, STPs have 75% out of 44 which support SP. This can include dance, music classes and singing as well as other things. There are 207 CCGs, like you said its made up mainly of HCPs. If in your opinion, we have more people involved in the STPs with people from the art sector, then those individuals can influence the decision made from an up down stream of information to try to include more services focusing on arts. What's your opinion on that?

Louisa – I mean I don't know enough about STPs, I suppose if they are involved in clinical prescribing then I think that sound like a very positive thing to invest more time and resources into this and to develop the links with the CCGs. I also think solutions could be diversifying CCGs so that you just don't have medical professional that sit on those group. Alternatively, some sort of process by which the LA can provide linking up with local organisation or some sort of process which can effectively gain access to the CCGs. I think it's quite touch and go depending on the locality and depending on the make-up of the CCG as to how connected they are to their community and what's happening in their community.

So yes, in principle, if the STPs are really active in supporting SP and if they were giving further resources to have more profile and more weight to encourage medical professionals to be looking at SP more seriously and looking at better ways to allow that to happen within their area. I think that's a positive thing. I will consider it further.

Arun – Have you heard about the NHS 5YFV? So yes, this is what got me into writing this book and which inspired me to raise the awareness of SP and digital prescribing (DP). Like when we do an SP service, it's in collaboration with the CCG, Health & Wellbeing Board (HWB) and LA. So essentially, an art practitioner or dance practitioner may be able to join the HWB, have you heard of them before?

Louisa – Yes, we have one here actually. I am not on the board, but I have been to some of the meetings to access some funding through the HWB local assembly. We have local assemblies in the Borough which have small pots of money. I think part of the issue is the complexity of the system so even the fact we have a HWB, the CCG, the LA, all of it is very complex and it doesn't necessarily need to be but that's just how it all evolved.

Arun – I think what's happening lately, since the inception of the NHS, is how to quantify the improvement in health and wellbeing parameters for participating in a dance activity or arts-based activity. One of the things which could be addressed is with IoT and wearable trackers like the FitBit and Apple Watch. Think of having up to 200 devices at home which are connected to the internet and providing real-time data and it's going to become the norm in 2020 when 5G get launched.

One vision of mine is when a participant does a dance class and has his or her health parameters measured in real-time, and afterwards you can see actual improvement with numbers, not just qualitative feedback by quantifying the measurements. This would be providing a better case for the NHS to fund art-based activities. I was just curious to hear your opinion on this subject.

Louisa – Yes, we have a dance science department here at Trinity Laban. The first dance science department that was created, so we have done various measurements both quantitative and qualitative and mixed methodologies for measuring impact on varying population of participants. We have considered the FitBit type approach particularly in relation to a group we run for adults who have acquired brain injury or stroke. One of the main issues with that population is a lack of access to accessible physical activities and therefore there tends to be very low levels of activity in that population.

There are high levels of obesity in that population, so any increase in activity levels both from taking part in class and even outside the class itself is positive. Our hypothesis is that through taking part in the dance session, participants have been more active in their normal day to day lives because they feel more confident and so on. Yes, we had many discussions with the science team about using those as a way of measuring, we used varying other measures, focus groups, surveys, standardised questionnaires, using different verified scales.

Generally, what we found is that they are not particularly successful in telling us the true impact of the work itself. I think what's problematic about trying to use medical measures is that the expectations with lots of those measures in the health world is that you are working with very large sample size in order to be able to show significant impact. Whereas in an art context, the number of participants that you are working with comparatively is much less so actually, you can never show the same amount of significant impact as you can in a medical trial.

So, I think potentially sometimes as an art organisation, we spend a lot of time trying to fit into a medical approach to measuring impact on our participants. When actually, the richness of what's happening for those participants lies in the stories and the qualitative responses of them as opposed to the numbers or the tick-box exercises. I fully understand, from working with the health world over the last 5 years that talking in their languages is really important, so mixed methodologies are the way forward and I know that FitBit would greatly support that.

This is because it's much richer/accurate in terms of the data it captures than a survey or any kind of measurement. However, I still fully advocate for the more qualitative/creative approaches to research in this area particularly within dance in health. At the moment, we have some funding from Kings' Cultural Institute to work with the same group with brain injuries that I described. We are conducting a series of different interviews/focus groups and our researchers are going to be about writing up what the participants perceive the impact of the dance classes to be. I think in a sense that perceived impact is almost just as more important than the actual quantitative measurements on what the impact is because if they think they are more balanced, if they think that have more strength, that's half a battle.

I do think evaluation and research is very important and I think FitBit could be a great way without being too intrusive or without using reductive measures which I think don't capture the richness of the activity or really ascertain what the true impact is on the participants. I think it also makes you look at things in isolation. We did a measure once called "the timed get up & go", we did it with our physiotherapist and basically you get timed from when you are sat in a chair to standing up to reaching and grabbing a ball and coming back sitting down and they time you.

It helps you see whether you have improved in relation to your strength, core stability, balance, that kind of thing. However, when looking at the results from this in isolation, it's a bit limited. We can just say yes, the class is supporting a greater core stability etc, but there is so much more going on than that. It's not just about core stability, it's about confidence, engagement, relationship building, there are lots of other things that go alongside that get lost when we just stick to very just standardised measurements. For example, that measure cannot tell us that one of our participants can now dry his back with a towel because of our class.

Arun – You have given me a new idea, have you heard of brain exercises? Like BrainHQ, which is a set of exercises developed by Dr Michael Merzenich who is a leading pioneer on neuroplasticity. By doing BrainHQ, it provides you with quantitative results on your ability to perceive a certain activity like the speed of your reflexes, the ability to see simultaneously moving objects and it kind of quantify the improvement over time. One of the idea I had last year was to combine BrainHQ with dance classes to improve your body's function, to become stronger, an improved core stability and doing the brain exercises to improve your ability to remember more dance moves which act in synergy more than anything.

What's your opinion in combining both for improving both the mind and body function as well as creativity?

Louisa – In a sense, I don't think you need to because everything is already in your dance class if you are delivering a high-quality class. So, in terms of cognitive function, actually there is lots of research around how dance reduces the onset of dementia in earlier age because of how it improves/supports the neurological pathways. A dance class encourages you to use your memory, to explore and learn different patterns physically and cognitively, develop spatial awareness, the use of rhythm. So various aspects of a dance class are already supporting healthy neurological pathways and strong cognition.

I think dance is a very particular art form, it's very unique in that it is highly physical. Within an education context in the UK it sits within the PE curriculum as a physical activity (despite being an artform). It provides a robust 'tool box' to deliver useful, engaging, artistic activities within a range of contexts, for a variety of populations with varying needs. We don't necessarily need to combine with established physiotherapy exercises or established brain function exercises to achieve positive health and wellbeing outcomes. Let's look at what we already have within dance, and work on refining how it can be delivered, the approach, type of activities, creative, artistic, physical, choreographic content etc. to improve the health and wellbeing outcomes for participants.

So, we should always look to our art form and everything it has to offer before we assume combining with other things will improve its impact. This de-value the art form unnecessarily. Not to say we don't learn from established exercises/existing research that comes from specialist fields, but I don't think we need to necessarily embed these things within a dance class. I think the tools we need are there already, it's just about the quality of delivery and careful design of that activity. Understanding exactly what are the needs of the participants and therefore the areas you wish to challenge and then designing the content of the session to support this. I think we have the potential to do that with this art form because it is both artistic and physical.

Arun – Do you have anything else you would like to add for pharmacists wishing to increase the uptake of dance classes for senior citizens, or for individuals who may be suffering from depression, anxiety, or even young people that may be doing self-harm from lack of confidence?

Louisa – Yes, I am a big advocate for dance for everybody, so I think everyone should have the opportunity to take part in high quality dance activity. I think certain types of dance, for me creative and contemporary dance practice, can support people who are living with all sorts of different conditions. I think assuring the quality of the delivery presents the biggest challenge. Making sure that the practice is delivered to the best standards and its meeting the need of the participants who are at the centre of the work.

In that respect, if the activity is participatory by nature, at Trinity Laban we ensure our practice is high quality by using the three basic psychological needs as a foundation; autonomy, competence and relatedness. So, all our artists try to achieve those things to ensure people are engaged and are motivated to continue to attend these classes. That's half of the battle – retention. I do think dance should be for everyone, it should be a way of life, anyone should be able to access dance at any point in their life whether they are suffering from a health condition or not. Dance is beneficial for everyone both physically, psychologically, creatively and socially. So yes, absolutely, it should be on prescription (Rx) but it shouldn't have to be on Rx, it should be a daily occurrence in everyone lives. But if it encourages people to engage with it then dance should absolutely be on Rx if it is high quality.

Interview with Alistair Spalding, Artistic Director and Chief Executive, Sadler's Wells

Arun – I was inspired by the Elixir Festival, could you tell me more about how it all started?

Alistair – Elixir was born out of the desire to recognise and celebrate the contribution to the art form made by older dancers, and to challenge assumptions about who can dance. Particularly in a professional sense, dancing is viewed as a young person's activity. There is a mistaken belief that by 40 or 45, your career is over. With the festival, we're promoting debate on whether this really must be the case. We aim to show the richness and benefits of creativity in later life and advocate for more work for older artists to be made and shared with wide audiences.

We believe dance should reflect and respond to the world around us, represent every aspect of it on the stage, including the diverse range of people making up our society, individuals of all ages and backgrounds. Older dancers may not perform the same, extreme physical feats of younger dancers, such as high-powered jumps and lifts. Instead, they bring something else to the art form, like quality of experience, nuanced interpretation, wisdom and confidence.

The other key objective of Elixir is looking at how we keep ourselves healthy and living well, and encouraging people to be physically and mentally active. In many ways, the festival is a continuation and development of our work with the over 60s. We have been running two successful initiatives for over 60s at Sadler's Wells for a long time: The Company of Elders and the Lilian Baylis Arts Club. Thanks to this track record, we've gained a reputation for offering high-quality programmes for older dancers and participants. Elixir was taking this commitment to explore and promote the benefits of dance in later life further.

Arun – As a pharmacist and krumper, I came across a video of Hip Hop-eration from New Zealand on Facebook in 2013. Then in 2016, I made the decision to write a book about pharmacy and dance since I am also a Dance for PD practitioner. Since there are many dance classes for seniors in UK, do you think there should be a platform for them to perform?

Alistair – Yes, it is important to offer work for mature artists a bigger platform. This is why, besides a conference and workshops, the Elixir festival features performances by both established dancers and community groups.

There are many ways to provide a platform for older dancers, from personal initiatives to presentations in institutional settings. People can create their own platform for performance in their community or town, and also be offered a stage as part of public events such as street parties or festivals. There are loads of interesting places where you can show what you are doing.

Arun – In terms of the NHS 5YFV, there are many pharmacies becoming HLP accredited. There are strategies set out for reductions in falls and increase the wellness of senior citizens. Have you considered to do a collaboration with Public Health England, to raise awareness of the Elixir Festival and to inspire the dancers who attend their local over sixty classes to perform locally or the following year? This could reduce social isolation.

Alistair – We're committed to raising awareness of the great benefits of dance to mental and physical wellbeing and are always looking for opportunities to do this, including working in partnership with other organisations.

In recent years, there has been growing public recognition of the benefits that engagement in dance brings to society, from improved mental and physical health to higher levels of educational prospects and civic participation. In particular, the government's announcement, in its new strategy for sport published in December 2015, that it was removing the previous distinctions between sport and physical activity, including dancing, was very encouraging, and confirmed the rise of dance's importance in the public health agenda. It was an official recognition of the effectiveness of dance and other physical activity in reaching under-represented groups in sport, such as people who may not consider themselves to be sporty, and not only helping them to be active and fitter, but also improving their general wellbeing, including by combating loneliness.

There is now an official push by the government and the NHS to encourage people to look after themselves better, triggered by the realisation of the vital importance of preventative strategies. We know that living a healthier life translates into needing less medical attention.

This is a welcome development. We need to fundamentally change how we think about our health and also about medicines and treatment. My wife is German, and the Germans are very focused on prevention rather than treatment, and it's a much better and cheaper approach.

In terms of initiatives at Sadler's Wells, besides Elixir, our Company of Elders and the Lilian Baylis Arts Club, we have been supporting Silver Routes, an over-60 community dance group that meets weekly at St Luke's Centre in Islington, as part of our outreach programme. We're currently working with social enterprise Breathe to present a performance in a healthcare space in spring 2018, when we're also going to deliver a series of Company of Elders Experience Workshops in our local community. And we are cultivating relationships with health organisations to hopefully be able to do even more in future.

Arun – Up to twenty percent of GPs visits are for non-medical reasons, so doctors haven't got time to explore the lifestyle of the patient for the appropriate referral which could be dancing, singing, cooking, walking groups and gardening so they use a Link Worker who is also known as a Community Navigator. This individual has a one-to-one conversation with the patient to find out their interests and what they would like to do, this empowers them to reduce social isolation. Social Prescribing Network (SPN) is the umbrella organisation of all social prescribing schemes in UK. Have you considered to frame Elixir Festival as part of social prescribing to help overcome the language differences between the arts and health sector?

Alistair – I wasn't aware of the SPN, but it sounds like a good vehicle through which to empower people to find a personalised solution and improve their wellbeing. Certainly, from our experience running the Company of Elders, we know that members don't just enjoy the health benefits deriving from the physical activity, but also very much value the social aspect of being part of the company, as their coming together regularly for rehearsals and performances makes them feel part of a family, less isolated and lonely.

Arun – Do you normally have a representative to go to the Age UK conference to talk about Elixir Festival, or is Age UK the only organisation you work with mainly?

Alistair – We don't currently have direct links with Age UK. There is an arts charity and social enterprise Aesop, which runs a falls' prevention dance programme called Dance to Health. They work in collaboration with dance organisations as well as health and social care partners. NHS England and Age UK are among their Dialogue Partner organisations. I have spoken to Aesop's founder and chief executive Tim Joss, and last year went to their conference at the Royal Festival Hall to launch the programme. They had guests from many dance and health institutions, including Simon Stevens, Chief Executive of NHS England. We are all trying to forge deeper links between cultural and health organisations.

We are also sharing best practice and actively participating in discussions with international colleagues about how arts and culture can contribute to elderly people's mental and physical wellbeing. Earlier this year, our Director of Learning & Engagement Joce Giles was invited to give a presentation on our work with older adults at the British Museum as part of the Age Friendly Museums Network Conference. He was also part of a working group organised by the Family Arts Campaign to develop their new age-friendly standards. More recently, Joce travelled to Japan with another Sadler's Wells colleague, three members of our Company of Elders and the company's rehearsal director in September, to discuss how the arts benefit the over 60s at an international conference held at the Saitama Arts Theater. They gave a presentation on Sadler's Wells' over-60s programme and delivered a taster session and dance workshops. Joce also took part in a panel discussion alongside David Slater, director of Entelechy Arts, which was chaired by Yoshiyuki Oshita, chief director of the Center For Arts Policy and Management for Mitsubishi UFJ Research and Consulting. The debate looked at how theatres' future programmes could focus on creative opportunities for elderly people.

Arun – Moving forward, where you do see Elixir Festival in the next five years? Do you think it will still be held in London or, similarly to Breakin' Convention, the festival will also tour to different cities and potentially different countries?

Alistair – There are no plans to tour Elixir at present, but we have been promoting how dance benefits the elderly through talking about our over-60 programmes and sharing best practice with colleagues at international conferences and events, as well as by presenting performances of the Company of Elders in various countries, including Austria, Italy, the Netherlands, Sweden and even Japan. Championing this cause is very important right now. We have an ageing population and dance, and the arts in general, bring demonstrable increases in wellbeing and improvements in health.

Arun – To finish off, do you have anything you would like to add for the readers who will be pharmacists on why they should themselves go attend the Elixir Festival? This could then change their perception on what a certain age group can do with their body.

Alistair – Pharmacists have an important role in patient care, as they support people in their communities on a daily basis and are able to provide valuable advice. I think that experiencing the Elixir festival would give pharmacists a sense of the tangible benefits that the art form brings to health and wellbeing so that, when engaging with elderly people, they could share their first-hand account of what they have seen and encourage senior citizens to take up dance as a way to take care of themselves by being more physically and socially active. The more we spread the word, the better.

Interview with Jennifer Neff from Elemental SP Software

Arun – In regards to your merge of your company with your current business partner, what was the reason? Was it the desire to create more social innovation or more like co-production as you both had the same vision?

Jennifer – Myself and Elemental Co-founder, Leeann Monk, have spent fifteen years working in community health in neighbourhoods across Northern Ireland. We've been the Link Workers, the program managers, we've run the community health programs, sourced the funding, issued funding and we've reported back to funders, so we know how difficult it can be.

We read a lot of the research and about the recommendations for the sustainability of social prescribing and its future. We knew all too well about the challenges in community health. We spoke with over 750 different stakeholders in community health from commissioners, providers, health and social care teams and most importantly the community. We found that the challenges around reducing health inequalities all stemmed from the fact that there was no integrated system to connect up all the key players in the health and wellness improvement supply chain. What was happening was that, despite everyone's best efforts, those that needed the most support were often being left behind.

We simply wanted to make it easier for people with health risks to access and engage in programmes and services in their community that would contribute to them living better quality lives. We wanted to arm those who are in regular contact with these people with the tools, information and the reporting ability to connect, support and measure the impact of the community referrals.

We wanted to provide the Voluntary, Community and Social Enterprise sector with the data to show the impact that their programmes and services were having and the difference they were making to people's lives, the community and the health and social care system.

We always say that SP is really the community development approach to community health. We believed so much in SP that we both gave up our full-time jobs and started Elemental. We knew we could make a difference to the sustainability of social prescribing and that digital had a major role to play in this.

We carried out our own research, which was evaluated by Ulster University and we knew that the responsibility of SP couldn't lie solely with the GP because of the pressures they're under. So, we saw an opportunity to work with the housing association sector and other sectors and we could see that they were playing their part in the health and wellness of their community, their tenants and residents.

Essentially, we are scaling, providing quality assurance and measuring the impact that non-medical referrals into the community. I think the key difference in particular is the ability to track the referral beyond the point of it being made and we have the data to show the individual and cohort journey. For example, an older person attends this particular be-friending service every week or a local luncheon club. Elemental identifies their baseline health risk and focuses on the person and how they are as a result of engaging in their SP choices. Elemental helps determine what difference has been made to the community and how it operates and what the impact is being made on the health and social care system now that this person is more connected, and their health risk has reduced.

Arun – In terms of social referral, one of the things that happened after coming back from the SP conference, there was a referral system on PharmaOutcomes called "Live Well Referral". I told the patient to expect a phone call soon. The following day, I received a phone call from the H&W team, I was the first pharmacist in Swindon to actually use the system and they were pleased. I asked them how long do they take to get in touch with the referred patient and they said that they can take up to three weeks. With your software, what's the timeline like?

Jennifer – It's all instant. We've made the initial referral process easy. It can be electronically in under 60 seconds. So once the referral is made, for example, it goes to the Link Worker and they can see straight away. The GP can check has the Link Worker made the call yet to meet with the person.

This was one of the problems that the GPs talked with us about, saying *"when I make a referral, how do I know it has been acted upon?"*.

We know how busy the link workers are too so wanted to facilitate their conversations with individuals and give information relevant to them. We have made their usage of the system really simple with instant referrals being made to a network of providers in the community and their referrals are all sent electronically.

Providers have access to the system also and so do the patients/ residents. It's all about making sure the individuals get the support they need.

Arun – Amazing, I wish we could do that more often.

Jennifer – If we could do this in pharmacies, that would be brilliant, and it would be something so simple to just be accessed by their staff on their screens. We're integrating at the moment with some of the GP systems so there is no reason why we couldn't integrate with the pharmacy system as well.

Arun – Definitely, I was able to refer three patients using the "Live Well Referral" on PharmaOutcomes. If people were using the services like yours which is instantaneous, then it would give an analysis of whether the patient has attended or not, this would be much more compelling for more pharmacists to take it onboard.

Jennifer – Elemental is enabling health and social care professionals to say, *"I made 100 more referrals this month compared to last month and here is the difference referrals are making to their health risk"*. They can track the progress of their initial referral to make sure that it has been activated. They also told us they wanted to see the risk reduction of the individual and the group of people they referred.

Arun – Exactly, when I was speaking with Denise Shelby from Doctors 2.0 & You conference series, she mentioned about multi-channel marketing. She was saying that if you wanted to deliver a message to a patient, just doing it with one technique may not be enough. At the time of writing my book, I always thought to keep social and digital prescribing separate but once she said that I was like why not integrate them both together.

For example, like in Sweden, it's quite common for estate agents to use VR for clients to look at the property before making the decision to purchase it. So, you don't have to physically go to the house to view it as everything is in the video. I said to myself, surely if you could bring this concept into pharmacies, especially in small cities where there are no link workers or a H&W team, you could have VR videos of each activity to help them make a decision like *"I want to do gardening", "I really want to try dance classes"* without having to physically go to that class.

You will just speed up that time, so what is your opinion on the application of VR for social prescribing referrals?

Jennifer – Definitely, we would love to really take it to a whole new level and we would really be interested and partner up with someone to explore that whole AI side.

We have our roadmap for our future design of the software for the next eighteen months. We have a list of things that we have on there and it's all determined by need and demand at the moment by those commissioning, delivering and receiving social prescriptions.

Arun – When I was at a King's Fund event, there was the CEO from Snap40 who made a device which fits on patients' biceps in hospitals. For deteriorating health parameters, a signal is sent to alert the doctor on duty, so they can see that patient. During the Q&A, I said that it was great that you could see a drop in their baseline and asked about the reverse, as in improvement in health parameters and he said that he didn't think about it.

What is your thought on a wearable tracker which measure the health parameters of the individual before they attend the social activity and after. So, on top of the social isolation score, you will have quantitative evidence that their blood pressure was reduced, his oxygen saturation has improved as a result but just wearing it for the session, they don't have to wear it all the time.

When you mentioned AI, it can analyse the results to look at the improvements ever since the referral to the link worker. In my opinion, this would attract many more stakeholders because they prefer when quantitative results are available. This was the impression I was given when I was trying to convince them to take SP onboard.

Jennifer – Technology plays such a major role in scaling and measuring the impact of social prescribing. We are all about testing new approaches, we've always been very evidence-based focused and we are all about partnering up to explore new and innovative ways to engage communities in their health and wellness. We welcome the opportunity to talk to people about the future of SP.

We've worked in the past two years with the Dubai Health Authority in the United Arab Emirates building the ecosystem for social prescribing to tackle type 2 diabetes. We carried out research in 2016 in Dubai and we found that people are ready to make the lifestyle choices required to reduce the development of conditions like type 2 diabetes. Their big ask of us was, 'We know the risks, help us to prevent' and that's what Elemental is doing.

Interview with Denise Silber from Basil Strategies

Arun – From your background in Digital Health, you give lots of motivational speech. In pharmacies, we get limited interaction. When we give people advice on doing more exercises, having a healthier diet, we only have one conversation for the whole year (I am referring to MUR) for the patient to take it onboard.

Motivation could be managed through a mobile app, such as by tracking a daily intake of calories or achieve goals to lose weight by exercising. What's your opinion on the concept of digital prescribing and the prescribing of mobile apps to patients to assist them when we do a consultation in the pharmacy,

Denise – There are different layers to your question from my experience. There is the question of what motivates a person to change their behaviour, how to put this into practice, and which tools to use. All of this must be aligned.

Hybrid methods work better to convince somebody in a long-lasting way. This is what is behind "Multi-Channel Marketing", for example. If we want to succeed with some big national public health issues such as smoking, overweight and proper nutrition, in getting people moving, we need to do much more than before. We need to mix use of the apps with contact with the pharmacist, for example, who enquires about the patient's progress.

This brings us to the issue of whether the pharmacists and the consumers have access to the same electronic file. The holy grail electronic file has often led to the downfall of digital tools. Either we hear about the NHS difficulty in connecting all the data or the issue of sharing personal data and signing consent forms. "Blockchain" is a very recent technology that is presumably going to bring trust to the sharing of data, because the history of the data cannot be modified. But the proof of concept remains to be developed.

The issue is really matching the goals of the pharmacy and pharmacists with the goals of citizens. If the pharmacist must spend gratuitous time, these projects will not succeed. The issue is that humans have contradictory motivations. That is why we're seeing unhealthy behaviours. So, programs have to be really well thought out and then gamified.

There has to be some incentive that makes things enjoyable. In driving, there is a negative incentive on making mistakes, because you can damage your vehicle, it can cost you money, they can take away your license. And it would be even better, if there were positive rules such as the better you drive, the more money you get back from your insurance or maybe you even get points to attend dance class!

There is research showing that pharmacists in communities have gotten together and decided to attack diabetes or smoking in Asia, Europe, and the US, and it works. However, I have never seen a national, run by the government kind of operation, a program by pharmacists that really scaled up. The largest one I have seen is in the US where Walgreens offer people the possibility, 24/7 to chat with a real pharmacist, who alternates between working in the store unit and responding to chat conversation. I don't believe these online pharmacists are doing prevention programs, but they are facilitating access to a professional.

Ideally, there would be one platform on which all the consumer's activity with the pharmacy, whether in person, or online would be found.

Another challenge is that unfortunately, the people that we most need to reach are the least pro-active. Why isn't there a mechanism by which the pharmacist can be reminded and contact such a patient? It would be easy enough to set up.

To summarize, a lot of people think, like you, that the pharmacist is in an ideal position because they are accessible and not in as hierarchical relationship with the consumer as would be the doctor.

However, if the pharmacist is already squeezed for time, and they aren't going to get paid, and there is no consumer platform, and the goals haven't been set, there is a huge gap between theory and practice.

Arun – In the UK, there is more emphasis on social prescribing which is referring patients to non-medical activities like gardening, dance classes, meditation for people that may be suffering with their mental wellbeing.

Denise – What is the incentive for each party?

Arun – We are regulated by the General Pharmaceutical Council (GPhC), the incentive for pharmacists is to follow a number of standards which include *"Make the care, health and wellbeing of the patient of our first concern"*. If we just provide medical advice, we are meeting the standard for medicines and health but we are not covering the wellbeing aspect which, is part of our ethical and professionals responsibilities.

One of the incentives is to meet the objective set out by the regulatory body for their health and wellbeing. For the patient, it is to get better thanks to deprescribing, i.e. that they can reduce the number of medicines taken. This was highlighted at an SP conference where two patients became empowered to take ownership of their H&W and were able to reduce the medication they had to take. One accessed his medication record and the other attended arts classes. They are both giving speeches nationally to share their story and the importance of patient empowerment.

Denise – It takes twenty-one days to form a good habit, if it is done at the same time every day, until finally it is routine. Let's take mindfulness. Nowadays many people are convinced of its usefulness, but it's good to do it at a set time, such as when you get up, or before you go to bed. However, so many people get up in a rush to get out and at night, are just too tired. So, they have very good reasons not to do it, unless they are in a mindfulness camp or retreat.

Arun – There is an app called Headspace.

Denise – Yes it provides ten sessions for free but then, you have to pay a monthly fee, which for many people would be out of reach.

Arun – There is a charity called Anxiety UK who offer a free twelve months usage of the Headspace app, as they formed a partnership. Hopefully, by that time, they would have learned how to do it without using an app. Regarding multi-channel marketing, I was thinking of using one or the other but I didn't think to combine the both of them where it would make so much more sense.

Denise – A good conversation with a pharmacist can go a long way, but it must be private, even if in the pharmacy. *"OK, Mr Smith, how would you like to proceed? How will you follow up on the prescription and recommendations? Would you like some help? Would you prefer a chart on paper or to use an app on your phone?"*

The pharmacist needs to have various options at his disposal. And the client's decision may not be definitive. They may start with paper and switch to an app.

Arun – Since there is an increased trend to use wearable trackers, it would be great if we had a device that is specifically made to facilitate messaging between the pharmacist and his or her patients. When I was speaking with one of the empowered patients, he wanted to record the conversation during consultation, listen to it afterwards, and share it with a caregiver.

Denise – Many years ago, there were start-ups in the US that proposed recording conversations between physicians and patients. They never scaled up. People may be readier for this now.

Arun – Yes, we have SCR as read-only access in pharmacies. There are plans to roll out a version which will enable us to add entries there. Potentially, future release can include a version for patient access.

Denise – This remind me of "Open Notes", which refers to the fact the physician writes notes about the consultation and the patient sees them, which is new. You could do the same between patient and pharmacist and provide that human touch.

Arun – There is an ongoing debate on the human touch being lost as automation becomes more prominent in various fields including AI. There could be a time where the pharmacists and doctors won't be needed anymore, as AI will be making all the decisions for the patients. What's your opinion on this subject?

Denise – The jury is still out on that one. It looks everyday as though AI is becoming more powerful in making decisions. But, if there is a major error provoked by AI in health, even though it could be due to a human programming error, I don't know if AI would recover.

We don't know that much yet about AI's capacities. People were hugely surprised that AI could work in the game of GO, because it is so multifactorial. And yet the AI program that did that doesn't have general ability, beyond GO. While AI is great for fields where there are known patterns, every day in science and medicine in general, we have to be ready to manage pivots. The human discussion will be important to flesh out the algorithms.

I know we are going faster than ever but much of everything we are doing today is already twenty to thirty years old. They were trying to develop various forms of connected glasses in the 80's. We see many things in science fiction, but we are still not there yet.

Some people say *"Look, we now have an artificial pancreas"*. But how many people could we put on it? A diabetes specialist cannot look at all your numbers of insulin, see a true pattern and give you a proper recommended dosage. People always think the weather tomorrow is like the weather today, because they can't make sense of ten days of weather, and they can't make sense of ten days of insulin either.

So yes, you would be better off with a program that can take into account many numbers but for human behaviours, you cannot yet reduce it to a number.

Arun – Essentially, empathy, the human connection is a crucial part of the consultation.

Denise – Thank you for bringing that up. We met on LinkedIn and you and I are having a good conversation. We are getting the best out of each other, even though we are not in the same room or even in the same location. And that is amazing!

Interview with
Eugene Borukhovich
from Bayer

Arun – Should entrepreneurship programs be offered in every School of Pharmacy (SoP) in UK to enable pharmacists to be inspired to lead start-ups in PharmacyTech?

Eugene – Yes, I think entrepreneurship across all program is required. Specifically for Pharmacy, indeed the dynamics, the patient & health consumer journeys are changing with technology advancements. So, what worked for pharmacies for centuries may not work in the future. Entrepreneurship courses can teach aspiring pharmacists on a different way to approach and identify the current challenges.

Arun – Like Hackathon, should a similar contest be run between SoP to generate moonshot thinking and disruptive ideas? The most innovative one could then be offered access to an incubator/accelerator program.

Eugene – Hackathons are just part of the tool-belt and touches on culture more so than identifying a specific need and hacking it. I am a huge fan of hackathons because you can think without constraints to find solutions but then quickly turn on the time constraint, to just get stuff done. It's a good way to identify some talented students who could potentially, not just do things better, but do better things for the patients and consumers. Certainly, moving the best outputs into further incubation is a good logical step forward.

Arun – Which is the winner between precision medicines and behavioural analysis (e.g. biohacks)?

Eugene – I strongly feel it's not a "winner" concept. Citizen Science has taken hold with people "hacking" their bodies and tools to help them understand. As these become more and more prevalent, especially in the rare disease space, the industry will adopt these approaches towards personalised medicine. I don't want to define personalised medicine here, but I would also argue that it needs to be personalised health. Ultimately, us, the healthcare consumers want and need health as an outcome and not medicine.

Arun – What's your opinion on Universal Basic Income to help move citizens from a scarcity mindset to an abundant one to improve mental wellbeing?

Eugene – This is still a philosophical discussion and given some pilots going on in the Nordics and other places I am curious to see the outputs. Personally, I am a fan but human nature, unfortunately, is also rooted in shirking. So UBI needs to be rooted into trust, how we ensure this trust is the philosophical part.

Arun – When do you see value-based care become mainstream across NHS services, including pharmacy?

Eugene – To be honest, I have stopped following the NHS since changing roles but if I take this to a broader global level, this needed to be done yesterday. Back to my point earlier, whether we as consumers pay for healthcare today via cash, private insurance or taxes, we want to see results. It involves extending and improving the quality of our life with family, friends and loved ones. There are many obstacles in the way, but companies like Outcomes Based Healthcare are paving the way starting in the NHS.

Exclusive Interview with Blockchain Expert

I had the huge privilege to do an interview with Rajesh Dhuddu who inspired me to launch PharmacyCoin to connect all the knowledge gathered from the 23 highly insightful interviews with world experts.

This is a preview on the information which will be discussed in my second book in collaboration with two other health futurists. The interview needs to be read after you become familiar with the principles of social and digital prescribing so that you become enlightened on the limitless possibilities with Blockchain and other disruptive technologies.

I highly recommend watching his TED talk "The Blockchain Revolution" as this is like the Internet in the 1990's. By getting involved now, you will be able to make profound changes for the pharmacy profession and leave a legacy for the future generations of pharmacists to come.

Interview with Rajesh Dhuddu from Quatrro

Arun – Blockchain could be used for dispensed medicines in pharmacy where entry in the ledger cannot be altered, and can also be used for over-the-counter medicines like cough mixtures to monitor potential abuse.

Rajesh – Basically, Blockchain will help to avoid the misuse that you are mentioning. It will give people visibility like an audit of purchases made by people. This is not only in documenting such trail of purchases, but also transmitting the information with the people in the network and it has to be correlated to previous medical history of that particular person.

Then you can make an informed decision that the person is buying this medicine for genuine use or for abuse. Having said that, I don't think Blockchain is the only technology that is available to be able to accomplish this. The key point is in terms of how easily you can transmit all information both current as well as historic to all participants in the value chain, so that they are empowered to make a correct decision. This can be accomplished by other technologies as well but the question has to be contemplated whether Blockchain is easy to implement, or if an alternative one is easier to do so.

At this point of time, we do not know fully the cost of implementing a Blockchain-based solution, but logically it appears that Blockchain is a lot more suited a technology to make information immutable or tamper-proof, especially for deployment of solutions in a public network.

Arun – Also, there could be a Pharmacy Passport where Blockchain networks can be accessed from a different pharmacy to allow streamlining and monitoring of medicine usage (e.g. asthma inhalers).

Rajesh – Absolutely, that's a very good goal. You can use the passport to basically see the history of the medicine's usage. Number one, it gives a good visibility of the patient history. Number two, it can provide authenticity of the requirement of a medicine. Number three, it can be used in the proper utilisation of the resources because in the UK and other places, the government pays for everything, it's a big social benefit that is available to the citizens.

Government is also to ensure that the people who are rightfully eligible to such social benefit. From a business case perspective, from a need perspective, it's very good but as they say, *"the devil is in the detail"*. Also, how do you implement it and how do you ensure that all the information is put into the Blockchain network, or any equivalent network? If I understand, especially in Western countries, people want to closely guard their information, it's like a personally identifiable information (PII).

People don't want easy access to that information, they consider it as very intrusive in nature. You need to basically come up with measures which will incentivise people to change their habits. So how do you incentivise people to change their social habits in terms of sharing their information in a timely basis, one needs to think about it. That challenge will be there, even if it's a Blockchain technology or not. I think such changes in the intervention of behaviours can be facilitated by an appropriate educational program, by an appropriate incentive structure or by an appropriate peer advocacy. So for example, I have a set of friends and three out of five of them have adopted, then officially I can get motivated to adopt and internalise change.

The biggest thing is that technology is available to bring in this change, also the choice of technology is available but how do you motivate or bring about the change in the behaviours, that is the key aspect of it.

Arun – We could use social prescribing where the ledger can add an entry when the patient attends the gym or yoga class as part of the agreed plan with the pharmacist, it can be reviewed at the next meeting when they collect their medication.

Rajesh – They may feel that there is no need for the network to know about what's happening in their lives. It can include going to the movie or restaurants. The social behaviours are completely different. You need to find out who the early adopters are, like those who like to write everything about their life and share information freely. Not because they want to show off but they want their network to know what they are doing, how are they living, what are they accomplishing and related aspects.

Number one, they must be willing to share information about their daily life. Number two, you must be clear on which parameters to share, like from a smart watch, and who will have access to that data. To turn that data into an insight which then can be an action point. I will give you an example. In one of my visits to Dubai, I went for a morning walk in the park and there were government officials asking people to enrol in a health program. It was targeting obese Arab nationals and getting their weight checked at that point of time, and they were asked to take a challenge. It was to either walk in this park every day or exercise daily and after a month, whatever weight they shed, they would multiply it to an equal ounce of gold and give it to that person.

Let's say you have lost a certain amount, I will not give a kilogram of gold, but I may give you one ounce of gold for each kilogram lost. The government is doing it because in Middle East, they have social benefits, there are no social benefits for immigrants. However, they were targeting both groups as there will be peer advocacy and pressure on the local citizens to take part too, if immigrants join in the program.

If two people are local citizens and they signed up, they would have accomplished their tasks of advertising to at least two nationals and reduced the overall government spending on the healthcare benefits of the national. This is so that spending can be diverted to something else which is more useful.

Arun – Yes, the UK has one of the highest percentages of obesity in Europe. If we had a similar scheme running in UK, there would be many people becoming more slim.

Rajesh – Yes, also in the UK, you don't directly charge for healthcare benefits, it comes from taxation. If you have to bring behavioural change and with the technology like Blockchain, you can use that healthcare information of people with good & healthy habits; it may have a positive effect on their rates of taxation.

Arun – Wow, that's a mind-blowing concept.

Rajesh – Exactly, I lead an active life, so the government are spending less on healthcare benefits. So, why should I pay the same taxes rate as another person who doesn't lead a healthy life. I am basically funding another individual by paying equal taxes.

Arun – It reminds me of people on benefits; some people get upset over the fact that they have to work to get paid whereas the others don't and still get paid.

Rajesh – Yes, this is fine, because if you don't take care of unemployed people then the crime rates increase in society. However, why should I pay taxes for somebody who has unhealthy habits and I take the burden of those particular taxes. I think progressing economies and progressive societies over a period of time supported by the appropriate technology, will get over it. I think it will happen over a period of time, it's not magical, it may sound like something out of fiction but I guess when equitable justice and appropriate governance mechanisms are in place, they will catch up with things. All those interventions must come with it.

Arun – Yes, especially with the fact that the global population is getting older.

Rajesh – Absolutely, your healthcare spending is going to go up because longevity of life is going up. You cannot always pay for taxes right after one stops working. Let's say I stop earning and I turn sixty years old, I may live up to eighty so for twenty years, I am not paying taxes but I am getting benefits. It may not impact government spending in countries like India because government doesn't fund the healthcare but in countries like UK, it becomes a huge burden on the government.

Arun – Thank you so much for opening my eyes. My vision is the integration of IoT to Blockchain, like wearable trackers which can measure iron levels, ECG, oxygen saturation, pulse rate, sugar levels and blood pressure to help the doctor or pharmacist recognise alarming results or trends which may not show up at the consultation (snapshot rather progressive monitoring).

Rajesh – The number of years is not dictated by technology but by adoption. I will give you an example, the current crime rate can be controlled by installing video cameras all over, like in the UK, through that you can control the rate of crimes by allowing investigations to take place. If you come to India or Sri Lanka, show me a number of roads which have video cameras installed, it's very limited. Is it because there is no technology? Is it because it's not affordable? No, the technology is easily accessible to these countries as much as the technology is accessible to Western countries. This is because you don't want to adopt.

My point is if you don't want to adopt, even if you have technology which is available at the click of a button, you are never going to solve that problem. Number one, I think adoption is important. Number two, there must be an appropriate governance structure from the government to push the adoption. Even today, there are IoT devices like Smart Watches that are available, they are affordable, but let's say, how many people in your family uses a smart watch that monitors heart beat and calories to help one take corrective measures. The price is around fifty pounds and is affordable for some members in your family. However, not everyone adopts it.

Arun – You are 100 percent right.

Rajesh – The problem is people don't want to internalise it. You may want to gift it to your father and he may not use it because he doesn't see the value in using it. Whereas, if somebody said to you, you will use it because you see a phenomenal value in using it. So the difference is he is not able to internalise it whereas you are able to. The focus should be on internalisation in addition to making the technology available.

Arun – Yes, this would work well in synergy with an incentivised program like the Dubai one. An increased perceived value will increase the internalisation process. Another possible application is patient medicines return with unopened boxes taking advantage of shared economy to reduce fees paid (unless they are exempt on prescription charges) by supplying it to another patient who takes the same medication, rather than going to the pharmacy for us to dispose of it or even supplying those same returned medicines to developing countries where access of medicines is scarce.

Rajesh – I think that's a very interesting concept. For unused medicine, they will become expired and will need to be disposed. There is technology available where you can put a RFID (Radio-Frequency Identification) tag into every box of medication. Based on a motion study, if the boxes are not moved around, it means nobody has touched it, it remains in the shelf unused and you can detect that. You can reach out to those persons to ask for their help in returning the medicines.

It will help you accomplish one hundred percent enrolment in this initiative. I think humans have always survived using the concept of recycling surplus items to those who are in deficit; that's how humans have survived. This applies to both developed and underdeveloped countries. You need to have a facilitating factor to build this. I call it a combination of cutting edge technologies and a large behavioural change.

Arun – Is there anything else you would like to add?

Rajesh – Yes, this may be an interesting observation for you to add. People should not be hung up on a participant technology. Blockchain seems to be the most preferred one from an implementation perspective and adoption in the peer-to-peer network. I think people should be more motivated by benefits and the best technology that is suited to promote it. They should be open to the technology whether it is Blockchain or a different one. All I am saying is they should not be hung up in trying to force a Blockchain technology to accomplish a benefit.

Join The Revolution

I hope this book has opened your eyes and allowed you to realise your full potential as a pharmacist, who is not currently utilised by the current system. Do use this book as a template to lay down foundations for Movement Pharmacy within your speciality or area of interest like singing, running and yoga classes.

The world is your oyster if you truly believe it. Engage with your entrepreneurial spirit, don't hesitate to network at non-pharmacy events to remove yourself from the echo chamber of negative individuals.

Surround yourself with people who uplift you and support your vision on what you want to achieve in your lifetime. To leave a legacy for the future generation of pharmacists who will follow in your footsteps.

If you enjoyed this book, please do read my next book on Pharmacy Futurism in collaboration with Denise Silber and Dr Xavier Schneider.

Like what Robin Sharma would say:

"Dream Big, Start Small, Act Now"

Made in the USA
Columbia, SC
18 January 2018